OUTBREAK BEHIND BARS

OUTBREAK BEHIND BARS

Spider Bites, Human Rights,
and the Unseen
Danger to Public Health

HOMER VENTERS

 JOHNS HOPKINS UNIVERSITY PRESS | Baltimore

Johns Hopkins University Press
2715 North Charles Street
Baltimore, Maryland 21218
www.press.jhu.edu

Library of Congress Cataloging-in-Publication Data

Names: Venters, Homer, 1967– author.
Title: Outbreak behind bars : spider bites, human rights,
   and the unseen danger to public health / Homer Venters.
Description: Baltimore : Johns Hopkins University Press,
   2025. | Includes bibliographical references and index.
Identifiers: LCCN 2024035207 | ISBN 9781421451435
   (hardcover ; alk. paper) | ISBN 9781421451442 (ebook)
Subjects: MESH: Communicable Diseases | Prisons |
   Prisoners | Disease Outbreaks | Human Rights Abuses |
   United States
Classification: LCC HV8833 | NLM WA 300 AA1 |
   DDC 365/.667—dc23/eng/20241228
LC record available at https://lccn.loc.gov/2024035207

A catalog record for this book is available from the British Library.

*Special discounts are available for bulk purchases of this book. For
more information, please contact Special Sales at specialsales@jh.edu.*

EU GPSR Authorized Representative
LOGOS EUROPE, 9 rue Nicolas Poussin, 17000, La Rochelle, France
E-mail: Contact@logoseurope.eu

For Georgia, Anthony, and Drae
Our Alpha, Ace, and Sigma

CONTENTS

OUTBREAK BEHIND BARS

Germs and Jails

Why Outbreaks Are So Harmful Behind Bars

Dennis Oya started coughing in late 2019 in a Washington state prison and kept on coughing for a year and a half until he'd broken three of his ribs. In addition to his cough, Mr. Oya started having trouble breathing. "Every time I called home," he said, "you could hear me coughing. I couldn't get full 20-minute conversations with my family, because of shortness of breath."[1] Mr. Oya knew he might be suffering from tuberculosis (TB) because he'd been diagnosed with the infection as a boy, but when he reported his problems to health staff, he was tested for COVID-19, and when that workup was negative, he was assessed for having a hernia and allergies.

Mr. Oya would go almost 18 months before the health staff in his prison listened to him, conducted a test for TB, and finally diagnosed him with the treatable but deadly and highly communicable disease. His infection would trigger one of the largest prison TB outbreaks in decades. Like many people who contract an infection behind bars, he didn't worry just for himself but for the people around him too: "There are plenty of other people around me who were put in danger.

Like my cousin—got tuberculosis. One of my other cellies: he got tuberculosis because of me."[2]

This TB outbreak would march across two of the state's prisons and infect 25 people. In order to map out the extent of the outbreak, the Centers for Disease Control and Prevention (CDC) and Washington health officials identified over 3,000 people who were close contacts, including staff and incarcerated people at five different prisons, as well as incarcerated people who'd returned home.[3] Although 25 people were identified as contracting pulmonary TB from this single case, a total of 244 contacts appear to have contracted a latent TB infection, meaning they didn't have any known prior exposure to TB and now tested positive. In these cases of latent TB, the bacterium is somewhere in a person's body, but it's not causing a lung infection—yet. About 5–10% of people with latent TB will develop TB infection at some point in their lives, most often in the two years after exposure.[4]

TB is a good model for learning about outbreaks behind bars because the disease is the leading infectious cause of death worldwide, and it's basically a disease of poverty.[5] Rates of TB are usually higher behind bars than outside, with a recent study showing worldwide rates are 10 times higher in prisons than within local communities.[6] In the United States, jails and prisons have long made an effort to screen people for TB, but the ways these systems fail illuminate the structural weaknesses of correctional health during other outbreaks.[7]

Case Study Analysis

Two problems stand out with how Mr. Oya was treated. First, the prison he was in already had a policy to recheck everyone for new physical signs and symptoms of TB annually. This is a standard practice in jails and prisons, and it includes an encounter at each one-year mark of incarceration to ask a series of questions about TB, including whether or not an inmate is experiencing night sweats, cough, weight loss, fever or chills, and several other potential symptoms.[8] The epidemiologist who wrote about Mr. Oya's case, Dr. Katharine Walter, reported that these yearly checks weren't happening because of the strain of responding to COVID-19. There is no doubt COVID-19 outbreaks in jails and prisons caused extreme spikes in illness and death, and increased pressure on medical systems. And when a health system is overwhelmed with an emergency, it might reasonably delay some types of encounters. That isn't what happened with Mr. Oya, though. He simply never received his TB check, and it wasn't until he developed symptoms of the disease and agitated for many months on his own behalf that he was finally tested.[9] This is what I see most often in jails and prisons: when scheduled medical care is delayed, it gets forgotten or cancelled until the patient manages to effectively raise the alarm.

Delivering care behind bars is a constant exercise in interruptions for many reasons: patients aren't brought to clinic, bringing medications to housing areas gets interrupted, or transports to outside clinics and hospitals get delayed or cancelled. These obstacles are so common that a standard task for the people who run a health service (and those who monitor from the outside) is to track how often these interruptions occur and record their causes, including lack of correctional officer staff (to escort the medical staff), lack of medical staff, security events like lockdowns, or even weather- and power-related incidents. Often, these delays turn into cancellations or rescheduled appointments, but very rarely do the administrators in these settings have the ability or approval to track all the delays in care and then make sure they are addressed. Tracking delays so they can be addressed makes sense if the goal is to deliver care or prevent morbidity and mortality. But if the goal is to avoid getting in trouble for these delays, then the health service (or the security service that controls them) may not want to have records of this problem. For a health administrator working hard to ensure patients are connected to care, the lack of adequate security staff is a particularly difficult issue, since tracking and reporting on this may annoy or anger the security service for whom they work.

The second failure that stands out in Mr. Oya's case is even more alarming: he couldn't get the medical staff to pay attention to his insistence that he needed a TB test based on his self-reported symptoms of the disease. While patients can be ignored in any health setting, there are special forces behind bars that can lead correctional health staff to disregard or disbelieve their patients. This can occur because there is a general cultural attitude among prison staff that being incarcerated means you are not credible in a general sense. This kind of neglect can also stem from a lack of adequate staffing to respond to anything outside of obvious emergencies and whatever the health staff want to focus on. As a review of other outbreaks will show, people who are incarcerated often report—both in writing and verbally—the exact symptoms of a disease to health staff, only to be disbelieved or ignored. This lack of response to new symptoms causes a delay in treatment for the person seeking care, but it also widens opportunities for the infection to spread to others, from incarcerated people and visitors over to staff and their families.

Of course, the spread of TB from Mr. Oya to those around him was facilitated by the physical nature of prison. Few human spaces promote the transmission of disease better than jails and prisons. Some of the reasons for this are obvious, like the physical layout of facilities. Other factors are more hidden, like the lack of basic health services and disregard for critical data if it comes from incarcerated people or runs counter to the facility narratives. The history of outbreaks in these settings, from tuberculosis to skin infections and viral outbreaks like COVID-19 and influenza, shows that many of our most basic tools and protections go ignored behind bars, and that, without fundamental changes, these facilities will continue to experience outbreaks that harm the health of incarcerated people, staff, and surrounding communities in preventable ways.

Examples of What Works

Communicable diseases are pathogens that jump easily from one person to another. These types of infectious organisms have natural allies in the physical design and operational neglect of prisons, jails, and detention centers. From TB to staphylococcal skin infections, bacterial meningitis, and COVID-19, correctional facilities can jump-start outbreaks, both large and small. Outbreaks in jails, prisons, and immigration detention settings are not rare, but because the health care and outcomes are kept hidden, the general public rarely hears about them. In addition, public-health officials are usually involved as a last resort and often without any meaningful oversight about how their recommendations are implemented or maintained. As a result, outbreaks of disease enabled by close human contact and lack of hygiene and sanitation, and made worse through lack of access to health care, wreak havoc behind bars.

Arrest can promote outbreaks well before a person arrives in jail or prison. After police arrest someone, they transport them to a local precinct and place them in a crowded holding pen with others, where they may sit on a bench or lie on the floor and share one toilet for up to 24 hours. This process can transform a single infection into many. People usually spend hours in these pens, then they make their way to a court arraignment, where they wait in another pen, then meet their lawyer and sit in court while a judge makes a decision about their bail. After this type of in-person arraignment, detained people either go back to jail or are free to go home. Some jails rely on video arraignments, which can reduce the contact of recently arrested people in court pens, but this option keeps these same people inside jail pens until they are either released through bail or held awaiting their trial. Some of the first contact investigations I took part in involved people who came through the New York City police and court holding pens and then were diagnosed with or even died from meningitis. In 2019, the US Border Patrol placed a 16-year-old boy into a holding cell despite the fact that the child had already been diagnosed with the flu. His story became well known when he died in that same cell, lying in a pool of blood. Shockingly, he was only discovered because of the intervention of another detained person.[10] The Border Patrol did not report on any additional infections resulting from close contact with this young man, but it seems likely the preventable death he endured led to other infections of those around him.

A 2018 pneumococcal outbreak at the Ventress Correctional Facility, an Alabama state prison, illustrates how overcrowding is a potent accelerator of outbreaks behind bars.[11] Pneumococcal disease is caused by the bacteria *Streptococcus pneumoniae*, which can result in infection that ranges from mild respiratory illness to pneumonia, sepsis, meningitis, and death. This bacterium is spread by respiratory droplets, and unlike many communicable diseases, an effective vaccine exists that can prevent it, which is especially important for older adults and those with compromised immune systems. The Alabama prison system became aware of the outbreak when three incarcerated people at the Ventress prison became ill enough to require hospitalization—one of whom died after suffering meningitis.[12] The CDC and the state department of health were called in to assist with the investigation once the cause of the infections and presence of an outbreak were established with blood cultures. In their review of the outbreak, the CDC noted that the original capacity of the six-dormitory facility was 650 inmates, that the capacity had somehow been "adjusted" to 1,650, and that the current census recorded over 1,200 inmates at the time of the outbreak.[13] The overcrowding in Alabama prisons is among the nation's worst, and three years later, during COVID-19, rates of overcrowding would still be a serious problem, including at Ventress.[14] The CDC ultimately identified a total of 40 cases of pneumococcal disease among the residents and staff of this prison, far greater than the 3 that were apparent to prison staff from the initial hospitalization.[15]

While there are inherent risks of outbreaks behind bars, there are also ways to reduce morbidity and mortality. One mitigation measure is to reduce the number of people who are incarcerated. This cuts down on crowding and quick transmission, and was used with success in the public-health response to COVID-19 (see later chapters). Being incarcerated creates multiple health risks, including infection from communicable disease as well as physical and sexual violence. The United States leads the developed world in our rate of incarceration, and this practice is heavily weighted toward Black, brown, and poor people. The work of Michelle Alexander, Mindy Fullilove, and others studying the prison system through a social-justice lens has been instrumental for me in coming to grips with how entrenched systems of punishment and racism and policies like the War on Drugs have led us to our current situation.[16] Abolishing our mass incarceration system is a broad and important movement that involves increasing investments in housing, health, education, and employment.

Reducing outbreaks behind bars may seem peripheral to this discussion about abolishing mass incarceration, but the issue shouldn't be ignored. There is sometimes tension between the two concerns, but learning the truth of conditions behind bars is critical to gaining support for alternatives, especially when we look at correctional settings as drivers of outbreaks. In addition, it's incorrect to think the risks from outbreaks (like those from physical or sexual violence) can't be addressed for incarcerated people. Being honest about the health risks of incarceration also requires being clear about how and whether those risks can be reduced. Returning to Mr. Oya's case provides good context. Had Mr. Oya been tested as required, or even tested when he first reported his TB symptoms, the smaller scale of the outbreak would have resulted in fewer infections and far less use of staff time and other resources. By comparison, a recent outbreak at a facility in Pennsylvania involved three men with active TB. All three patients were identified in their initial days of detention, and the contact with other detained people or facility staff was minimal.[17] The adherence to infection-control policies in the Pennsylvania facility had a concrete impact in reducing infection transmission for staff and incarcerated people. This one step—testing people for TB as they enter a facility and again each year—is a core CDC recommendation, but many of the places I inspect delay or miss it altogether.

This book provides another important lesson from other outbreaks: the impact of incomplete treatment. Every chapter here will present cases that were identified but then forgotten or ignored, leading to more transmission, morbidity, and mortality. When I started working at Rikers Island, there was considerable lore and pride about the role the jail system's communicable-disease unit played in turning the tide of New York's drug-resistant TB epidemic in the early 1990s. Between the late 1970s and the early 1990s, the number of people with TB in New York City nearly tripled, and many of these new cases involved drug-resistant TB.[18] Because a disproportionate number of these cases were identified in the city jail system (as well as other New York jails and prisons), Rikers became a focus of efforts to find and treat people. These efforts included a court-ordered construction of a communicable-disease unit with dozens of negative-pressure cells, state-of-the-art sputum-induction booths, and TB experts from the city's health department.[19] From my perspective in the New York City Department of Health and Mental Hygiene, these efforts by the TB control bureau were a kind of high-water mark for the agency and propelled many public-health professionals to the highest reaches of the field, including leading the CDC. These were truly important efforts, but almost lost in the historical context of this work is the basic link between the emergence of drug-resistant organisms and treatment interruption.[20] People with infections who are also struggling with unstable housing, substance use, incarceration, or lack of food or employment face an uphill battle with continuity of treatment, especially for medication regimens that stretch into weeks or months. This link between resistance and treatment interruption is true for many more infectious agents than TB, including viruses like HIV and hepatitis C, bacteria like *Clostridium difficile* and *Staphylococcus aureus*, and fungal infections like *Candida auris*.[21] Behind bars, treatment interruption is commonplace for medications like insulin as well as for antibiotic, antifungal, and antiviral medications. For patients with anything from TB to MRSA and scabies, when initial doses of medication stop arriving on the medication cart or in the clinic, there is often no system to detect these treatments have been accidentally stopped or delayed. This problem is almost as serious as the lack of initial detection, but the solutions require competent health administrators, with the systems to detect treatment interruptions, who are supported by the facility security leadership and, when needed, outside health departments.

If there is a unifying theme in what works during outbreaks behind bars, it comes down to listening and paying attention to incarcerated people. This sounds like an overly simple thing to do, but the barriers between incarcerated people and existing health surveillance and care are numerous and sophisticated. Incarcerated people's verbal reports to nurses and correctional staff may be ignored, and even written sick-call slips and emails sent from facility kiosks may be deleted or thrown away without action or review. The voices of incarcerated people can be tuned out in such a way that they almost disappear, despite the presence of many systems that are supposed to do the opposite.

Conversely, when outbreaks are adequately responded to, the success is often directly because of information or ideas that come from patients themselves. This is true for both large- and small-scale outbreaks. During COVID-19, one of the most successful interventions was to release people who were near the end of prison sentences and didn't pose safety risks, especially if they were at high risk for dying from infection. This approach was proposed by family members of incarcerated people and groups like the FAMM (Families Against Mandatory Minimums) foundation and the RAPP (Release Aging People in Prison) Campaign even before infections started moving across the nation. The idea was eventually adopted by the Federal Bureau of Prisons as well as many state prison systems—a move that saved lives and did not cause an increase in crime.[22]

When a facility finds itself in the middle of an outbreak, one of the most useful tools I've come to rely on involves conducting town halls in housing areas that have been isolated. There is often an effort to sequester, quarantine, or somehow isolate people in affected and unaffected zones during an outbreak. Inside each of these spaces, rumors and panic can quickly take hold, so it's essential that health staff visit the housing areas and both provide information and take questions. These settings can also have special processes in place to screen for symptoms and provide care related to the outbreak, as well as regular medical and mental health care. Speaking with people in their housing area is essential to understand how well these new workflows are being implemented. Outbreak-specific infection-control measures might need to be followed, such as social distancing or wearing personal protective equipment (PPE). But walking into a housing area and announcing yourself as a doctor, nurse, or public-health staffer who is there to answer and ask questions about what is happening sometimes reveals deep levels of distrust and anger, especially the first time it's done.

These meetings often start with people airing their grievances about the lack of health care or information about the outbreak, which is usually justified in my experience. But this type of discussion quickly yields important information about who is sick, what the real conditions of sanitation and hygiene are, and whether the efforts to set up surveillance, treatment, and prevention are working. It's also one of the few scenarios where correctional officers in the housing unit can learn and ask questions informally, away from their peers. In these discussions, the officers often reveal themselves to be caught in the same cycles of disinformation as the detained people. Whether tackling MRSA, legionella, *Clostridium difficile*, H1N1, scabies, or COVID-19, this kind of town hall is a tool that has served me and others well because it allows for learning and sharing information at the same time. During an investigation, additional efforts are needed to conduct confidential interviews, but in terms of day-to-day health services, success or failure during an outbreak is often linked to how well staff listen and respond to patients.

Before jumping into the following chapters, I need to provide some more context about the places where these outbreaks occur. The intended audience for this book includes people in public health, medicine, nursing, and other health professions. My expectation is that most readers will have little or no experience working behind bars. Two themes run through many carceral systems that bear on outbreak response: brutality and mistrust. Regarding brutality, it's a common (but not universal) feature of these facilities that physical and sexual violence are wielded as tools of control, intimidation, and retaliation. As I write this chapter, a horrifying story has emerged from an Alabama prison, the same system where the pneumococcal outbreak was fueled by overcrowding and so woefully under-detected. A 22-year-old man named Daniel Terry Williams died of trauma at the prison the day he was due to be released home. His family report he'd been beaten and sexually assaulted for days until he was finally taken to a local hospital. There, he was found to have injuries all over his body and no meaningful brain activity.[23] Aside from the devastating impact of violence on victims, their families, and survivors, violence and aggression also stand in the way of accurate information about how extensive an outbreak is. For example, I was taking temperatures in a high-security housing area during an outbreak at Rikers when five or six people jumped the person I was assessing. He was sitting at a metal table with the thermometer in his mouth, and I was next to him with a stack of screening forms and my stethoscope. When the other men jumped him, I grabbed my filled-out forms and stood against the wall as the assault played out, watching as the correctional officers initially tried to stop it with handholds, then turned to their pepper spray. Most nurses, physicians, and mental-health staffers who work behind bars have been in multiple scenarios like this, but I was only a few months into my time at Rikers, and this experience left me wary about how to work inside housing areas. I don't think all detention settings have a uniform level of violence. In fact, when I confidentially interview people, they report a wide spectrum of brutality, ranging from very little beyond the occasional fistfight to daily physical and sexual assaults that are not only tolerated but even directed by correctional staff. In the facility where the man I was screening was assaulted, I learned shortly thereafter that correctional staff in the building were both conducting and directing beatings of detained adolescents.[24]

The second theme relevant to preventing and responding to outbreaks is mistrust—which flows in almost every direction behind bars. This mistrust is driven by a disconnect between the official rules of the facility and the actual conditions under which people work and are incarcerated. Less distance between these two perspectives yields more trust, for sure. Causes of this mistrust can include a staff perception that patients submit frivolous requests for care and grievances about their care, while patients think their basic requests for care go ignored. Another source of mistrust revolves around short staffing, which can pit the patients, facility staff, and facility leadership against each other as services and access to care are limited. The presence of contraband in the facility and the unequal efforts to prevent or detect it among visitors and incarcerated people compared to finding out what comes in with staff is another area that can foment mistrust. The mix of these problems is unique to each facility, but they can combine to create a system where the official policies and procedures about health services are disconnected from reality. As a result, the access to and quality of care can be far removed from what we might expect in a hospital or outpatient clinic.

Another deep-rooted source of mistrust behind bars, especially toward public-health teams, relates to experimentation on incarcerated people. The unethical use of incarcerated people as human subjects in research is a modern problem. For example, in the 1960s and '70s, when the US government wanted to learn more about the effects of radiation, they contracted a doctor named Carl Heller who exposed inmates in the Oregon prison system to beams of radiation on their testicles.[25] At about the same time, researchers at the University of California San Francisco's medical school were exposing thousands of prisoners to pesticides and herbicides by placing the chemicals on their skin and injecting it into their blood.[26] Similar experiments were conducted into the

1970s on mostly Black men in Holmesburg Prison in Philadelphia by Albert Kligman, a physician would go on to develop the acne treatment Retin-A.[27] In the wake of these experiments, significant reforms were made to how ethical standards should be applied in all research involving incarcerated people. Now the need for people behind bars to be included in ethical research isn't in dispute.

A recent example of mistrust of health staff based on fears about experimentation occurred in an Arkansas jail during the COVID-19 pandemic. A jail doctor decided to treat detained people infected with COVID-19 using a potentially harmful and unsupported treatment, ivermectin.[28] About 250 people were given the medication, and a group of them filed a lawsuit as a result. One person in the jail said, "It was not consensual. They used us as an experiment, like we're livestock."[29] A judge involved in the lawsuit found that people weren't told they were receiving this potentially harmful and unsupported medication and that jail patients were given higher doses than those the physician gave patients in his community clinic. "Dr. Karas documented his Ivermectin experiments on social media. He admitted on his clinic's Facebook page the voluntary participants in his 'clinic regimen' received lower doses of Ivermectin as compared to his unwitting 'jail patients.'"[30] This doctor was hailed as a hero by local officials, and the Arkansas State Medical Board took no action against him.[31]

In the dozens of town-hall meetings I've conducted during outbreaks, I think experimentation and mistrust of the health service has come up in about half of them. This concern is especially prevalent when discussing vaccination or treatment with medications that aren't commonly understood (like antibiotics). Similar to the deep issues with physical and sexual violence, questions and worries about experimentation come from very real and harmful abuses of incarcerated people and can't be swept aside or ignored.

Mistrust of health providers behind bars is a case of patients adapting to their reality, but the mistrust doesn't likely stop when people go home. If anything, adapting to discrimination or neglect in health care behind bars is something that can impact engagement with health care after release. This phenomenon is directly relevant to outbreak responses since there's a predictable and regular need to offer screenings or treatment to people after release. In Mr. Oya's case in Washington, among the approximately 3,000 people who were identified as close contacts of someone with active TB, about 800 went home before they could be told about their exposure or screened for TB.[32] The work that public-health departments had to undertake to contact these 800 people and convince them to return calls and get screened couldn't have been easy and was undoubtedly hampered by mistrust of health-care professionals, especially when the initial ask was to delve into their experiences in prison.

Mistrust between the health and security staff can also be a problem, and it reflects failure in management as much as imbalances in power. I've worked in plenty of settings where the security leaders valued the ability of the doctors and nurses to make independent assessments and viewed their medical mission as something that shouldn't be infringed on. When this is the culture and attitude of security leadership, it shows. Conversely, when the basic requirements of seeing patients in a timely manner aren't present, it's usually because the security leaders don't value the mission, or because the health leadership won't advocate for their mission. Or both. I showed up to treat patients in a clinic one day at the New York

City jail barge and noticed that another doctor there wasn't seeing any patients. When I asked why not, he said, "The officer took my chair, so I can't see anybody." This seemed both insane and ridiculous, but after checking with the other staff and speaking to a captain, I found it was true that an officer had swiped the physician's chair and that this sometimes happened and became a reason patients weren't seen. The doctors need a chair to do their work, but this was my first introduction to the many scenarios in which health staff sometimes stop doing their work when it's interrupted by security staff, who run and control the facility. This was a jail clinic we operated directly as the city's department of health, not one being run by a for-profit company, so it was our own bad management and communication with security that had allowed this to happen. Over the following years, this jail became the site where I would see patients and bring medical residents for electives, and where our nursing leadership made important strides in improving health service. But still, the little ways in which a health-care operation can be subverted or interrupted when the health and security staff don't work well together are mind-boggling, with patients caught right in the middle and paying the price for these malfunctions.

How Chapters are Organized

Each chapter in this book includes some of the effective measures I've observed and learned from health and security staff in facilities I've inspected. These steps to prevent, detect, and respond to outbreaks are lifesaving, and the staff who implement them deserve credit for applying public-health measures in a way that not only reduces mortality but also decreases illness, pain, and suffering during outbreaks.

Each chapter will end with a few bullet points of recommendations and at least a couple of research ideas for public-health students and professionals. My intent with this book is to highlight some details about how outbreaks occur behind bars and how morbidity and mortality can be minimized. The list of recommendations in these chapters range from the big picture, like releasing people instead of incarcerating them, to the granular, like handing out biodegradable laundry bags and eliminating co-pays for medical care. I know that some of these recommendations are in place in some jails, prisons, and detention settings, but I've included them because they are relevant to morbidity and mortality, and they're also lacking in deficient systems.

Recommendations

- Jails, prisons, and detention centers should include infectious-disease treatments and other needed follow-up in their discharge planning encounters, which are meetings to make sure health services are set up for people before they return home. This follow-up would include a review of all people who were identified as having been exposed to TB but who didn't have pulmonary infection. They would need referral for treatment to prevent any latent TB infection from developing into a full-blown case. This work would also include a review of any people with pending contact investigation encounters.

- TB-related encounters in carceral facilities (and entire systems) should be tracked and reported to the facility and system quality committees. These reports should include the percentage of initial and annual TB assessments that are conducted within expected time frames.

Research ideas

- Hypothesis: People with latent TB infection are not consistently offered or started on treatment during incarceration. Approach: Examine the number of people with positive TB skin or blood test in jail who qualify for, start, and complete treatment for latent TB infection. Examine contact investigations by departments of health to see how or whether they extend to local jails, prisons, and detention centers. Review lawsuits that may provide information in this area.[33]

CHAPTER TWO

Spider Bite or Staph Infection

James Malles was detained in a Pennsylvania jail when he noticed a bump under his arm.[1] He was worried about developing a skin infection because he'd seen another person on the unit with large suspicious boils on his back, scratching his back on the shower wall. At the time, up to 14 men in his unit shared the only working shower. He'd heard that the man with the boils and others had been diagnosed with the skin infection MRSA (methicillin-resistant *Staphylococcus aureus*).

A few weeks later, Mr. Malles felt an itch in his right armpit and mentioned it to a nurse during the morning medication line on his housing unit. He took the last place in line so he could stay away from others and so he could show the bump to the nurse when his turn came. The response he got from the nurse was that the bump was probably caused by the water. Worried about infection, he started to wash his shirts himself in the small sink in his cell. Many incarcerated people have reported to me that they do this when infections occur and when they don't trust the laundry machines. In this case, Mr. Malles kept reporting his problem over the following week, morning and evening, to other nurses who came to his unit to dispense medications.

Time after time, when he reported the growing, painful bump under his arm, Mr. Malles was rebuffed with excuses and given no care. Responses included that the bump was nothing, that he should submit a sick-call request, that the water was causing the bump, that the laundry soap may have caused it, and that he should simply "keep on trucking." When he asked for a sick-call slip to write down his problem, he was told by one nurse that they weren't available. Over four or five days, one bump progressed to several, with a rash in between them. Ultimately, the bumps became boils that started to burst and drain fluid. Once the boils burst, a nurse finally did take him to a medical isolation unit, where a culture confirmed he had MRSA skin infection, which others already in the isolation unit also reported having.

Case Study Analysis

Mr. Malles's infection was part of a series of MRSA cases in this facility, and he did exactly what the policies in the facility called for, reporting any new skin rashes or boils to health staff. But as his case shows, getting people to report signs or symptoms of infection isn't much use if the health staff don't respond promptly to figure out the source of the problem and slow the spread of infections.

While COVID-19 and TB provide examples of how communicable diseases can quickly overwhelm jails and prisons, most outbreaks behind bars are smaller and may go unnoticed beyond the people who are directly impacted and their families. One prototype of this form of outbreak is skin infection from the bacterium *Staphylococcus aureus*. This bacterium lives on the skin of humans, but in conditions of poor hygiene and close quarters, a single isolated case can turn into a slow-rolling disaster, with scores or even hundreds of cases developing over a period of weeks and months. One of the deadliest of these infections is methicillin-resistant *Staphylococcus aureus* infection, named for its ability to resist antibiotic treatment and cause rapid illness and even death. The CDC gives a typically brief but terrifying description of MRSA: "It is found in the nose or on the skin of many healthy, asymptomatic persons (i.e., carriers) and can cause infections with clinical manifestations ranging from pustules to sepsis and death."[2] The CDC's photos of these infections are even more halting.[3] While MRSA has gotten some public attention during outbreaks in hospitals and other community settings, it represents a dangerous and ongoing source of outbreaks behind bars, even though much of the knowledge about these infections became widely understood and shared in the correctional-health field in the 2000s. Key tactics to prevent and respond to these infections include basic sanitation and hygiene in living spaces as well as active surveillance of all new skin lesions and boils with bacterial culture of any open wounds.

While a staph infection, including MRSA, can happen to almost anyone, outbreaks of multiple cases and transmission from one person to another most often occur in places where people share close quarters and some physical contacts, like the equipment in gyms and in hospitals. In the early 1990s, outbreaks of MRSA were well documented among high-school wrestling teams, with some athletes identified as not only experiencing skin infection but also being colonized with MRSA, which could pose a risk for ongoing transmission to others.[4] In hospital settings, MRSA and other staph bacteria present a well-known risk. In fact, the concept of hospital-associated infections is central to infection control and has been a driving force behind efforts to reduce mortality during hospitalization for more than a century.[5] The efforts to identify and mitigate health risks from hospital-associated infections are in sharp contrast with efforts, or lack thereof, in jails and prisons, where adverse health outcomes are usually attributed to the patient, not the place. Jail- and prison-attributable deaths are common, but the lack of transparency and accountability regarding these settings and the lack of involvement of the CDC and local health departments mean that rates and types of jail- and prison-associated infections (as well as virtually all other health outcomes) remain mostly hidden.

While some aspects of hospital and carceral infections may be the same, my own experience is that outbreaks of MRSA and other staph infections inside jails and prisons are largely driven by overcrowding, lack of hygiene that allows this bacterium to pass easily from one person to another, and a failure to detect and treat initial cases before the infections spread. Jails and prisons are places where official policies about access to showers, soap and water, and clean laundry may be ignored without scrutiny by any outside oversight group. These problems are especially true in areas shared by multiple people, like housing-area bathrooms, showers, intake pens (which may lack bathrooms and showers), and even places meant for health care like infirmaries and clinics. Most jails and prisons have a policy about the number of people who should share a shower or toilet, with ratios of one shower or toilet for every 8–12 people, but when I walk into housing areas of jails, prisons, and immigration detention centers, I often find these policies not being followed, with no consequence for the facility. Whenever I raise these issues, the reply I get usually refers to a recent construction project or issue with the plumbing, which makes the problems appear short-lived. But the reality is that most jails and prisons are decades old and the lack of adequate showering and bathroom facilities, as well as maintenance staff, is a normal state of affairs. In some of the places I've inspected, areas designed as holding pens (for short-term use of a few hours) are actually being used as jail housing areas, making the issues of sanitation and hygiene even worse. Similarly, the filthy conditions in these settings, with accumulation of food and human waste, especially in intake areas, are especially bad. These problems are often cleaned up before any planned inspection, so the few outside audits that occur tend to miss them.

A relevant problem reported by many incarcerated people is that care for skin infection may be initiated but then stopped prematurely, which can have a devastating effect on wound healing and prolong these types of infections. In the Northampton, Pennsylvania, jail, not far from where Mr. Malles was held, a very similar MRSA outbreak occurred in which detained people reported that "mattresses that had been defecated and urinated on were not cleaned or changed between inmates, and instead were quite often left in place for the next inmate's use."[6] One of these people, Mr. Demar Edwards, reported that while detained, he noticed a large, painful, discolored spot on his ankle. He was seen for this problem by health staff, who initiated contact precautions, cultured his wound, and started daily dressing changes—all good evidence-based responses. But after a week and a half, his care stopped, and his bandage was left unchanged for two weeks. When a nurse finally examined him, his wound was found to be "open," and the same precautions and treatments were restarted. The single lesion on Mr. Edwards's ankle spread into two wounds, and despite written orders to the contrary, he experienced more interruptions in his daily examinations and bandage changes over the following weeks. Months after his initial infection was detected, Mr. Edwards passed out and was transferred to the hospital, where surgeons performed multiple operations on his leg and ankle, removing infected tissue and even pins and screws from an ankle repair that Mr. Edwards had undergone years before his incarceration. While in the hospital, a pump was connected to Mr. Edwards's wound to remove pus and other fluids, and he underwent reconstructive surgery to graft skin from his thigh onto the area of his infection.[7]

In some cases, the contact between a person and their source of MRSA was even more obvious. In another Pennsylvania jail case, Mr. Kevin Keller reported that he was held in a cell for weeks with a person who had a large, open, and draining abscess on his back. Eventually, Mr. Keller developed golf-ball-sized boils in his armpit that also burst and started to drain purulent fluid. His sick-call requests went unheeded by health staff.[8] This case not only repeats the patient's inability to get care and treatment but also layers in the reality that incarcerated people face health risks in their housing, sometimes from violence or abuse, and sometimes from infection.

Unlike in community settings, the resolutions of these cases were not prompted by health departments or other legitimate health bodies finding these problems and forcing some improvements. Instead, incarcerated people had to find lawyers willing to take their cases and sue the facilities or systems where these infections occurred. The lawsuits were successful in that the counties involved were forced to pay financial settlements to the people harmed, but some of these people sustained permanent disability from their infection. And some of these lawsuits were brought by the families of incarcerated people because their loved ones had died. This kind of outcome—for a person to find an attorney willing to take their case, mount a successful lawsuit against a jail or prison, and then get a result that includes improvements in care—is extremely rare.

When I started working in correctional health in 2008, MRSA outbreaks were on my radar because of the huge outbreak that had occurred in the Los Angeles County jails and the lore about how the cases had been initially misidentified as spider bites. In 2002 alone, over 1,000 cases were documented in the nation's largest jail system. In the first eight months of the year, 57 people were hospitalized as a result of these infections, with some experiencing spread of the bacteria to their blood and bone, and requiring medication and surgical removal of affected tissue to save their lives. In the early days of the outbreak, detained people started reporting boils and wounds on their skin; both they and medical staff apparently assumed the culprit was some new harmful spider infestation. The jail medical director reported, "We spent a considerable amount of time screening all of our facilities, making sure that pest control measures were in place and actually trying to capture a specimen so we would have some idea what we were dealing with."[9] Once all the spiders that could be caught in the jails were sent to entomologists, they determined that the wounds were not the result of spider bites. Five months into tracking hundreds of cases of these wounds, the likelihood that they were infections from staph was finally established, and the jail started working with the county health department to obtain a wound culture on every new case. This effort started in June 2002 and resulted in identifying 928 cases. But as with late onset of COVID-19 testing, there is no doubt that many if not most of the cases that occurred earlier in the year were never accounted for, unless the people were ill enough to require hospital transfer.

The health department and the CDC would provide input on how to prevent these infections in the LA jails, including recommendations like regular access to laundry services and showers, educating detained people about the need to report these skin lesions, responding to those reports with speedy medical care and wound culturing, and keeping people with open wounds away from others. Two years later, the ACLU would file a lawsuit against the LA County jail system, reporting that many of these basic steps had not been implemented.[10] Specifically, the suit alleged the ongoing overcrowding in the jail had resulted in people sleeping and living in close quarters, as well as living in wet and dirty jail units, which left the interventions advised by the CDC and county health department unaddressed. By 2007, the total number of MRSA cases would rise to about 8,500, with no end in sight. By that time, a local mathematician, UCLA professor Sally Blower, would develop a mathematical model for predicting how the LA jail system served as a hot spot for MRSA, spreading infections to those who were incarcerated and, ultimately, out into the community.[11] This model, with the jail itself as the epicenter of infection, would gain little ground in terms of policy reforms but would become relevant once again with the arrival of COVID-19. But in the early 2000s, the model helped me to think about the jails as having their own risk profiles for the health of incarcerated people and staff, profiles that spanned risks from infections to physical and sexual violence, injury, worsening of chronic disease, untreated opiate and alcohol withdrawal, and, of course, death.

These two outbreaks surely are not the first, but they are crucial because they represent the point in time where the knowledge about the problem and the best practices for reducing outbreaks became widely understood. And thus, as outbreaks of MRSA and other staph infections persisted across US jails, prisons, and immigration detention settings, they occurred against a backdrop of indifference, not a lack of understanding. Because handling MRSA is such a core part of the CDC and local health departments' day-to-day work, multiple studies and best-practices resources to prevent MRSA and other staph outbreaks behind bars became widely available in the 2000s. In the wake of many specific outbreaks, including the LA County jail case, best practices were identified, including the need for shower access, laundry services, and cleaning of common spaces. These best practices also include educating staff and detained people about MRSA, the need to not share personal items, the need to report and quickly culture new skin lesions, and the necessity to implement medical isolation when there is a risk of transmission. But I regularly observe that these best practices around preventing, detecting, and treating skin infections are missing in jail and prison health care. These best practices also incorporate the health of correctional staff as a central component in preventing outbreaks.[12] This staff element is crucial in outbreak prevention and response, both because of the clout of correctional officers and their unions as well as the oft-overlooked reality that these staff move around facilities more than most incarcerated people, and so they act as primary vectors for the spread of communicable disease.

But as anyone who has recently stepped foot behind bars knows, many of these seemingly basic tools to prevent staph infections remain elusive. Laundry services may occur once a week or less, leaving people to reuse a single towel for all their needs. Hanging these towels up to dry may be a violation of facility rules, all but ensuring people are constantly using wet towels. One of the things people report when I inspect a facility is that hanging and drying their clothes and towels is forbidden because of the security concerns about blocked cell fronts and windows. In one recent inspection, the staff hadn't anticipated we would go to a particular housing unit, and officers ran just ahead of me, screaming at everyone to take down the towels blocking their cell fronts. Even when laundry services do occur, water temperatures may not be sufficiently high to kill staph bacteria. People also may be forced to use common hygiene items without any effort or opportunity to disinfect, such as having a single nail clipper for a housing area to use one at a time, or barber tools that are not cleaned or disinfected between uses. Every new MRSA outbreak seems to take facilities by surprise, as if the prior 30 years of national experience and guidance about prevention don't exist. Years after the CDC had reported on the LA outbreak and a similar one in Mississippi, a warden in a county jail said, "Back then, I don't think people knew as much about it—I had to learn about it when I came on."[13]

One of the core concerns about MRSA behind bars is the high prevalence of people carrying the resistant bacterium. We know that these infections can recur, and the risk factors for recurrence are both individual and environmental, meaning the likelihood of a person contracting an infection is driven by their own MRSA status but also by where they live or work.[14] Some people are colonized by MRSA after their initial infection, which obviously increases their likelihood of future infections, and sometimes, treatment to eliminate the bacterium from a person's body completely is undertaken after a second or third infection.[15] Between 10–15% of people entering jail settings are thought to carry MRSA on their skin or in their nasal passages.[16] While these estimates are from small studies, they reflect a rate many times larger than the general estimate of about 2% of all people being MRSA carriers in the US.[17]

The risks for MRSA are likely spread unevenly based on where in a facility a person is housed. Some of the worst conditions can be found in the facility intakes (pens where people are held for hours or days on the way in and out of the facility) and in the housing units where people viewed as problems are held, including solitary confinement and mental-health units. When I inspect these types of units, I often observe vermin, feces, and garbage throughout the living spaces. Violence and neglect are more common here than in other parts of the facilities, and the basics of hygiene are missing. I have investigated deaths in these types of cells, where people starved to death, were left after being seen eating their own feces, and were found dead covered in bites from vermin. It is a safe bet that whatever the approach to hygiene and infection control is elsewhere in a facility, if there are cells where people are locked in most or all of the day, those places are held to a lower standard.

In addition, COVID-19 has taken an immense toll on carceral settings, not only in causing direct infections among detained people and staff but also in decimating many of these basic standards of detention, like access to medical care and hygiene. The most public example of this is the disaster at

Rikers Island, in the New York City jail system. There, a combination of short staffing and managerial incompetence has led to people entering jail and spending more than a week in crowded intake pens, using plastic bags and milk cartons as toilets.[18] These people have been deprived of basic medical care, often because no staff existed to take them short distances for care. In other parts of the same jail system, short staffing has led to people with serious mental illness being locked in their cells for days on end. This may be the most public disintegration of a correctional setting in the United States, but it is far from the only one, and as people endure more squalor and less care in the wake of COVID-19, staph skin infections (along with overall morbidity and mortality) will rise dramatically.

Examples of What Works

So how can these outbreaks be prevented, especially given the ongoing reality that prisons, jails, and immigration detention settings continue to ignore very basic tools? First, it's important to reflect that many carceral settings have implemented some of these interventions reliably. For example, the rapid culturing of new skin lesions and even checking for skin lesions during the admission process are measures that I do encounter in jails and prisons, not uniformly, but they represent a very modest step that is achievable. Another effective tool is the use of standardized nursing sick-call forms for any report of a skin rash, lesion, or boil. These forms can be used in paper or electronic medical records, and they guide nurses, who are the ones most likely to encounter a new or emerging skin infection, through a protocol that includes wound culturing, notifying the infection-control team, using contact precautions, and referring to a physician. More challenging is the overall approach to showers, hand washing and drying, and laundry. Again, some facilities have a robust approach, but those that don't aren't likely to change simply because it's a good idea. And most challenging is the approach to over-crowding. Many state prisons have endured round after round of lawsuits finding them in violation of basic constitutional standards because of chronic overcrowding. But the threat of MRSA and other staph infections as they cram more and more people into small spaces seems like a very ineffective cudgel. As these lawsuits have revealed, MRSA is just one of the issues created by overcrowding, and even in less over-crowded settings, access to hygiene is often lacking—and access to diagnosis and treatment is absent.

All this points to the inconsistency and variability in how infection-control interventions are put in place. Without either a standard approach or public score card as we have in hospitals and nursing homes, we can be sure that many set-tings fall short of these basic approaches, and that people are becoming needlessly infected and dying from staph infec-tions. Unfortunately, lack of oversight and accountability is consistent throughout correctional health. In terms of out-break prevention and response, one of the most harmful impacts is that basic infection-control steps are only con-templated in the heat of the moment, and there is no pres-sure to maintain the staffing, skills, and resources once the crisis fades.

So these outbreaks of skin infections behind bars are a widespread problem, but what can we do about it? An impor-tant first step is for MRSA and staph infections to be in-cluded in the list of conditions that facilities are mandated to report to local health departments and the CDC. In the LA jail, many people initially went undiagnosed. That's a big problem, because not only do people's infections worsen without treatment, but there is also increased transmission to other detained people, staff, and families as people return home. In addition, by not tracking infections correctly, the appropriate level of health staffing, proper medication supply, and even the amount of space for safe numbers of people in housing areas go unexamined. Available data show that about 20,000 people die each year from these infections in the United States, but we have no reliable data reflecting all 7,000 jails, prisons, and ICE (US Immigration and Customs Enforcement) detention settings, where over 10 million incarcerations occur each year.[19]

A review of these infections in carceral settings in 2011 reported rates of MRSA roughly equivalent to community rates in some jails and prisons, while other jails and prisons reported rates 200–300% higher.[20] But their data was based on a simple review of a handful of places where cases had been publicly reported. Only a tiny fraction of the 7,000 jails, prisons, and immigration and juvenile detention facilities in the United States were examined. But we need to track these cases not just to understand the totality of the problem. We know that the genetic variants of bacterium isolated inside correctional settings are often unique, so the risk in ignoring these settings is that they serve as potent incubators of resistant infections. If we don't study these places, their infections could fly below our radar until people become so ill that they require hospitalization, creating a new opportunity for spread. If the CDC and local health departments start with the relatively mild mandate that correctional cases be reported to them, then they will be able to track rates of infection and show both the need for evidence-based resources and responses as well as the benefits of those responses occurring. Reporting these cases will also help reveal the ways in which the lack of other types of health services may contribute to MRSA, staph infections, and death. But the cases above also remind us that without a competent approach to correctly diagnosing these infections, reporting won't help much. Inside the lawsuit regarding the Pennsylvania cases mentioned above is an example of just how difficult it can be to find out that a patient has a skin infection, even when they have attorneys looking into their care. This account is from the counsel for a woman who had close contact with another woman who died after contracting a MRSA infection in the facility.

> She is a mental-health patient under care of CMHS and has recurrent staph boils from MRSA since early 2002, when she had daily contact with Virginia Brejack before her death in December 2001. On September 3, 2002 counsel spoke with her. She was getting no treatment and her attorneys were told she had no MRSA. On September 9 counsel obtained her medical records, which stated she suffered from "folliculitis," infected hair follicles. There was no report of testing for staph or MRSA in her file and no explanation for isolating her in solitary confinement. Counsel obtained laboratory reports via subpoena and identified Ms. Boka Smith's test as positive for MRSA. It was removed from her CHS file. After Plaintiff obtained counsel she was subject to retaliation, which continues. She has written numerous grievances requesting medical care.[21]

A recent death in the Naples, Florida, jail was identified as being caused by MRSA infection. But the man who died, Mr. Timothy Kusma, also had insulin-dependent diabetes, and experts have identified the lack of care for his diabetes and poor blood-sugar control as contributing to his death from MRSA.[22] This type of jail- or prison-attributable death involves two independent health risks from the facility: exposure to staph bacteria and inadequate care for a chronic disease. This combination of risks—the interplay between outbreaks of all kinds and chronic disease—is the topic of a later chapter.

After mandatory reporting of infections, a second needed improvement is to include skin infections and infection control in a basic facility audit tool for state and local health departments—not just for use during outbreaks but for yearly audits of health services in all places of detention. This improvement can be accomplished in a one-day facility inspection and can be combined with other health issues or conducted alone. Essential elements of this audit tool include understanding the following:

- Do people have access to laundry, showers, and soap?
- Do people experience skin lesions, and what happens when they report them?
- Do facilities culture and report skin infections as soon as they are reported, and do they monitor patients for recurrence and persisting symptoms?
- Are people housed in a manner that increases the risk of staph skin infections and other health problems?
- Do skin infections appear to worsen or be related to preexisting health problems?

This type of work requires more than sending a survey to jail or prison health staff; it must include speaking with currently detained people in a confidential manner. This approach also requires review of medical records, including sick-call requests, for people who do develop skin lesions so as to validate the information they and facility staff report. A detailed approach to conducting a facility inspection during outbreaks is in the last chapter of this book.

In many states, these improvements will remain out of reach because of a lack of public or state-government support. But in some states, like New York, there is an opportunity to grow this work based on what has already been accomplished. The New York Department of Health and Mental Hygiene has a legal mandate to oversee the adequacy of health care behind bars for HIV and hepatitis C care, and the arrival of a new governor and commissioner of health provides an opportunity to expand this requirement to other areas of health.[23] But even in states that won't take this approach, we can still push for mandated culturing and reporting of MRSA and other staph skin infections to local and state departments of health and the CDC. In many states, isolated MRSA cases are not reportable, and as the cases above show, an outbreak can smolder in a facility for some time before erupting. In addition, these cases make clear that a full-blown outbreak may occur without people being tested or treated, especially in short-stay settings like jails and immigration detention. Tracking records should include information about incarceration and not simply be a report from laboratories to these agencies. We have a longstanding appreciation of how hospitals served as early drivers of MRSA infections, and we must develop a similar focus on how jails, prisons, and immigration detention facilities can do the same.

Recommendations
- Jails, prisons, and detention centers should periodically compare sick-call requests and encounters involving boils and skin rashes or lesions with the

laboratory tests for wound cultures. This type of review can help detect instances when patients needed (but didn't receive) a wound culture.[24]

- Grievances relating to laundry, sanitation, and access to showers, sinks, and soap should be reviewed by the facility infection-control officer.
- An annual review of skin infections should be included in the facility quality committee's work.

Research ideas

- Hypothesis: Some people return home from incarceration with untreated sores and skin infections. Approach: Interview public defenders and recently incarcerated people about their experiences with diagnosis and treatment of sores and skin infections during incarceration. Review information from lawsuits in this area.[25]
- Hypothesis: Correctional officers may lack basic infection-control knowledge. Approach: Provide basic infection-control training with pre- and post-test competency questions for correctional staff.

CHAPTER THREE

Death and Disability from Outbreaks

B rett Fields was a healthy 24-year-old construction worker when he was booked into the Lee County jail in Florida in the summer of 2007. Shortly after arriving in jail, he noticed a small red sore on his arm and reported it to health staff. He received bacitracin ointment for his lesion, but it worsened. He tried several more times to seek care, eventually getting some oral antibiotics, but the boil on his arm didn't resolve. About two weeks after he arrived, he submitted a sick-call request about his skin lesion, but he didn't receive any response. He submitted another request 10 days later, reporting that the medications he'd been given for his open wound weren't working. Mr. Fields was transferred to a different cell for infection-control reasons, but he continued to deteriorate.[1]

One month after his arrival in jail, Mr. Fields noticed numbness and tingling in his back and legs. The next day, his legs started to twitch and spasm, and the back pain worsened. Mr. Fields and his cellmate hit the cell's emergency button to get help in the evening.[2] He testified at trial that he hit the button hundreds of times before a nurse came and told him he would have to wait until the next morning to be seen for the back pain and leg spasms. After the nurse had left and he continued to hit the emergency button, he was ordered by a correctional officer to stop. That next morning, court documents indicate that Mr. Fields tried to drag himself to the shower but collapsed along the way. As he dragged himself back to his cell, other people being held in the same housing area started to protest on his behalf, banging on cell doors and yelling for help. Eventually, nurses came, and Mr. Fields was put into a wheelchair and taken to the clinic. There, a physician assistant examined him. Mr. Fields reported that he couldn't walk and that he had pain and numbness in his back. An examination of his patellar reflexes showed no response to the reflex hammer hitting his knee; he similarly showed no reflex movement when the bottom of his foot was scraped. Somehow there was no recognition of a medical emergency, and Mr. Fields was given Tylenol and taken in a wheelchair to a new cell. Throughout the day, Mr. Fields reported to multiple nurses that his legs were weak, that he couldn't walk, and that he was in pain, but he was left in the cell. That night, he had his first bowel movement in days and experienced rectal prolapse, where part of the rectum slides and protrudes out of the anus. Alarmed, he and others in his cell block yelled for help, and a nurse came eventually. A court of appeals opinion in the case described what happened next.

> Mr. Fields explained that his intestines were coming out, and Ms. Allen demanded that Mr. Fields roll over. Mr. Fields, who was on the floor, explained that he couldn't move the lower half of his body. Ms. Allen jerked Mr. Fields' body, obtained some K-Y Jelly, and pushed the intestines back in.

Once she finished, Ms. Allen pushed Mr. Fields' legs back and forth. Mr. Fields, however, did not react.[3]

At 9:00 a.m. the next morning, about 24 hours into Mr. Fields's outright paralysis, a physician came in for a regular shift. None of the nurses that Mr. Fields had been asking for help mentioned him to the doctor, and after 90 minutes, the physician happened on Mr. Fields and asked him what was wrong. After a brief examination, the physician ordered that Mr. Fields be immediately transferred to the local emergency room. Nobody bothered to call for an ambulance for another 2 hours, but eventually Mr. Fields was taken to a nearby emergency department. There, physicians quickly ordered an MRI of Mr. Fields's spine, saw a spinal abscess that was putting pressure on his nerve tissue, and operated to remove the abscess that had caused damage to those nerves. Cases like this are true medical emergencies because patients who receive surgery and abscess drainage quickly (in less than 24 hours) are far less likely to have permanent damage to their spinal cord or nerves—which is unfortunately what happened to Mr. Fields. He would recover some use of his legs, but he would need a walker and braces to get around afterward, and he would have lasting bowel and bladder dysfunction. The judge in one part of his legal case summarized his condition by noting that "though Mr. Fields can, after years of rehabilitation, now travel with a walker, he is still partially paralyzed from the waist down."[4]

Case Study Analysis

Although the rest of this book focuses on the broad array of ways to prevent and slow outbreaks, this chapter examines how lack of diagnosis and treatment for infections can lead to death or disability. Mr. Fields's case, like some of the other MRSA cases presented already, shows how an acute infection can be incompletely treated, resulting in the infection never going away and actually spreading from the skin to other parts of the body. We often think of outbreaks in terms of mild short-term illness from influenza, COVID-19, or even staphylococcal skin infections. But, as we've seen, the deficiencies in detecting and treating acute illness during outbreaks behind bars can lead to death or disability. In Mr. Fields's case, his infection was apparent from his first day of detention, but the slow and ineffective responses of the jail health staff contributed to his ongoing infection as well as his risk of death, pain and suffering, and ultimate disability.

Mr. Fields filed a lawsuit against the for-profit company responsible for his care in jail, Prison Health Services (PHS).[5] His case went to trial, and a jury awarded him $1.2 million, finding PHS had been deliberately indifferent to his needs.[6] A crucial aspect of testimony from the jail's health staff established that aside from or in addition to any errors made by them, PHS had a policy of limiting care to save money.[7] The appeals court opinion in the case referenced the denial of care by PHS when rendering its verdict:

> Prison Health enforced its restrictive policy against sending inmates to the hospital. Ms. Allen testified that, at monthly nurses' meetings, medical supervisors "yelled a lot about nurses" sending inmates to hospitals. Repeatedly, Prison Health instructed nurses to be sure that the inmate had an emergency because it cost money to send inmates to the hospital. Ms. Allen remembered three separate supervisors who emphasized the policy to her.[8]

This same opinion concluded that

nurses, Ms. Allen said, "weren't trained to designate whether somebody" had "to go to the ER;" to the contrary, "that's a doctor's job to do." Hence, Prison Health allowed nurses to send inmates to the hospital only in an emergency, but then left them to figure out what an emergency was. To Ms. Allen, an emergency was narrowly defined as when someone is "dying any minute." Ms. Allen elaborated on her definition by giving examples of "emergencies." She, for instance, had called ambulances where a man was beaten half to death and where a man had no pulse, but had placed inmates with partial paralysis in an observation room.[9]

Cost pressures in correctional health can also impact the ability to prevent or initially detect infections. One of the most common areas where I see financial pressures manifest during outbreaks is the lack of infection-control staffing. Usually, a contract between a for-profit vendor and a county or state correctional agency will include some mandated infection-control staff. But when I've been inside facilities for inspections, I've often learned the role is unfilled and being assumed by someone who already has more than a full-time set of responsibilities.

Pressures to limit care based on financial implications aren't the only systemic contributors to disability and death during an outbreak. Another element affecting how infections can progress toward disability or death involves the patient simply not being believed by health staff. In Mr. Fields's case, court documents include the following harrowing account: "When she was done, Ms. Allen called Mr. Fields a liar. Ms. Allen stated that, if Mr. Fields had not gone to the bathroom for days, he would be in severe pain as she moved his legs. Mr. Fields explained that he could not feel anything below his stomach."[10]

Patients do sometimes feign illness, but when a provider suspects this is the case, they must obtain a very thorough history and conduct a rigorous physical examination. This is needed to ensure the patient's presentation isn't actually a serious problem or even a medical emergency (as in the case of Mr. Fields). This approach is also needed if the patient is in fact feigning illness, so that the health team can decide on the plan of care based on adequate details. For example, if a patient is thought to be feigning seizures, the health team should get a thorough history of the patient's seizure diagnoses, review community medical records and medication use, and possibly send the patient for consultation with a neurologist and testing via electroencephalogram.

My experience is that health staff often stop believing their patients when the doctors, nurses, and therapists accept narratives given to them by security staff stressing that a patient shouldn't be believed. This is very different from basing their perception on an independent assessment done themselves, and it's a common issue because of the pressure the security setting places on correctional health staff. The pressure on the health mission from security priorities is known as "dual loyalty," and it's a potent yet rarely discussed contributor to jail- and prison-attributable deaths. There is a powerful shifting of missions behind bars, whereby a health professional or even an entire health service can succumb to the priorities and opinions of the security staff, so that a patient with clear and objective signs and symptoms simply isn't believed. Dual loyalty pressures are omnipresent behind bars and, like infection control itself, must be actively sought out and identified.

When I worked in the Correctional Health Services of the New York City jails, we found that dual loyalty issues were most acute in solitary confinement and mental-health settings of the jails. When we engaged with staff and patients about these issues, they provided incredible details about how the health mission can be harmed or impacted and insights about how we could mitigate the potential for dual loyalty to harm patient care. With this information, we created a dual loyalty training module for all health staff that helped everyone learn about common scenarios involving dual loyalty and ways to mitigate its potential impact on care. These scenarios ranged from documenting injuries after use of force to ensuring access to medication among patients in high-security units. We published these trainings in a peer-reviewed manuscript so others could adapt them.[11] They were among the most positively reviewed trainings we'd ever had among health staff, with about 90% of participants indicating they wanted more of this type of training. We even turned the lessons into a continuing medical education module for the American Psychological Association, which was still active last time I checked.[12]

The problem of dual loyalty is relevant for outbreaks because security may already ignore or disbelieve people they are seeking to punish or who they think have a mental-health problem. In these settings, a patient could report or show textbook signs and symptoms of infection to a health professional and be ignored or disbelieved because the nurse, doctor, or therapist had already shifted their frame of the person's identity away from patient to something more aligned with how the security service viewed them.

In addition to the dual loyalty pressures that are concentrated in solitary and mental-health settings (and because of them), these physical locations are often more filthy and violent than general-population housing areas. People with acute mental-health issues are often confined to a locked cell all day. They may be allowed to come out for showers, some health encounters, and court, and thus have the potential to be exposed to many types of outbreaks. But back in their cells, they may not be seen or heard as they become ill, and their symptoms may be ignored or misinterpreted as symptoms of mental-health crisis. People who are in solitary confinement face serious barriers to assessment and care, especially when it involves having a confidential encounter with health staff outside their cell.[13] Health staff may come onto these housing areas briefly to give medications through food slots or quickly stop at the locked cell doors to ask about health or mental-health symptoms, in full earshot of correctional officers and other incarcerated people. As a result, being housed on one of these units can result in a steep drop off in a person's ability to seek or receive health services during an outbreak. It can also increase exposure to trash, feces, urine, vermin, and many other potential environmental sources of infection.

We learned about Mr. Fields's case largely because of court records. Most outbreaks or infections that lead to preventable disability or death won't ever take this path, and there also won't be any outside and transparent investigation by a department of health or the CDC. But when cases like Mr. Fields's do come to light, we often see similar features that involve a person coming to the attention of health staff early in their infection but being ignored or denied adequate care until their illness has progressed and the infection has spread. During this time, it is often other incarcerated people who are working to provide care and comfort, as well as raise the alarm about infections, the same way the people around Mr. Fields raised their voices and banged on doors to get health staff to see him.

I learned of this type of health advocacy among incarcerated people during many of my COVID-19 inspections. In a women's prison in Connecticut during the first months of the pandemic, I reported on a woman who was cared for by the women in her housing area:

> She became ill in the evening. No medical staff are present in the facility to respond to requests for assistance. She spent several hours in the bathroom toilet stall vomiting and retching, with several of the women in her housing area intermittently helping her. Some of them were also vomited on, they were not wearing masks or gloves. Later that evening or early in the morning of the 25th, a Lieutenant calls EMS and she is transported to the hospital where she is quickly intubated for respiratory protection, and tests positive for COVID-19. The next morning, other women are told to clean the bathroom floor where she was vomiting for several hours, without gloves.[14]

One of the first facilities I inspected was the notorious Metropolitan Correctional Center (MCC) in lower Manhattan. This facility had been plagued by multiple scandals before COVID-19, including sexual abuse of detained people by security staff and the suicide of Jeffrey Epstein while security staff were absent from their posts.[15] The development of COVID-19 at MCC appears to have involved (or coincided with) the presence of a gun in the facility. In late February 2020, officials received a tip that a loaded gun had been smuggled into the facility, potentially by staff, and a thorough search for it began, which involved transferring many detained people to another facility, then back again to MCC.[16] Following this upheaval, one person at MCC reported that his cellmate

> started to feel sick on March 23rd. I felt really sick too. On the 23rd, they took [name redacted] out and brought him back in twenty minutes and gave him some medication and told him he had a stomach virus. But he didn't get better. For three days, we tried to get medical attention again, but they did not take him out until the 25th. We had to bang on the door to get attention.[17]

At another facility I inspected responding to a COVID-19 outbreak, a similar effort to seek care for other detained people was evident. In Calhoun County jail in Michigan, one man submitted an electronic request stating, "Subject virus; Please check the people in this unit, many are sick fever, cough, headache, thank you." A response was sent the same day electronically, stating, "This request has been forwarded to the day clinic nurse. Thank you." At least some of the people in this unit had also reported their own symptoms to the health service but weren't tested for another week. This delay didn't only impact them; it also helped spread the outbreak because these people were "tray runners," people who took food trays all over the facility.[18]

Another hidden feature of outbreaks involves the extent to which deaths and disability are even attributed to the outbreak itself. I was asked by a federal judge to investigate the COVID-19 response in a Bureau of Prisons (BOP) facility in Lompoc, California. One of the people who died from COVID-19 in the very large outbreaks at Lompoc was Christopher Carey, a 72-year-old man. The BOP originally considered Mr. Carey to have recovered from his illness, but subsequent to his acute COVID-19 infection, he developed progressive paralysis and was hospitalized for several months before his death in December 2020.[19] His death was not initially attributed to COVID-19, but his autopsy report documented "Respiratory failure / Respiratory arrest secondary to paralysis secondary to COVID-19."[20] Even more difficult to track or attribute are deaths that occur right after release but which result from infection behind bars. The Marshall Project documented cases where men leaving prison settings with COVID-19 were not tested and died shortly after release. Among these cases was Mr. Alan Hurwitz, who was 79 years old and so infirm that he was pushed in a wheelchair by prison staff all the way to board a plane home. During a layover, though, the airline sent him to a local hospital with chest pains and a fever of 104°F.[21]

Examples of What Works

Mr. Fields suffered months of ongoing pain and illness as his MRSA skin infection made its way through his body and into his spine. He survived his incarceration but returned home with profound disability. Mr. Carey, the BOP patient who was reclassified as having died from respiratory failure and paralysis as a result of COVID-19, also endured many months of pain and suffering before he died. One of the first steps for anyone wanting to prevent or respond to outbreaks usually requires close examination of most serious cases of illness and death, but these cases may be difficult to find and understand. I recently attended a meeting of people who work to address problems in correctional health that included two leaders in this exact area of hidden deaths and morbidity. One is Andrea Armstrong, a law professor at Loyola University in New Orleans who has assembled a team of researchers that finds and documents deaths occurring in parish prisons. The other leader is Dr. Roger Mitchell, a forensic pathologist and the medical examiner for Washington, DC. One of the recommendations Dr. Mitchell (and others) have advanced is the need to include a box to tick on every death certificate that indicates when a death occurs in custody.[22] This simple change would allow us to know the most basic facts about who dies behind bars during and in the wake of outbreaks, and it would allow public-health officials and epidemiologists to examine deaths that weren't originally attributed to an outbreak, such as Mr. Carey's case.

Since the initial wave of COVID-19 infections in 2020, it has become clear this viral infection sometimes causes a wide range of long-lasting symptoms. Some of these symptoms are serious and debilitating, like shortness of breath, chest pain, and headaches; others are an annoyance, like loss of taste and smell. Some of the most common long-term symptoms I've encountered in meeting with incarcerated people include neurological symptoms, like ringing in the ears and fatigue. While these may seem like an annoyance, they can be debilitating in settings where noise and violence are pervasive, and where there is a mandate to work a prison job, or face punishment for not reporting to it, and to mix with others on a regular basis. For people who report these types of symptoms in a sick call, which often comes with a charge, there is rarely any appreciation that the symptoms reflect ongoing COVID-19 illness. There is also rarely any effort to arrange an appointment with a physician. While treatment of these long-COVID symptoms isn't always clear or effective, simply making the diagnosis is crucial, both for the person's benefit and for the institution to know how much new long-term illness there is from these outbreaks. People with preexisting health problems, especially heart, lung, and kidney diseases and neurologic disorders, will often experience worsening of those health problems after COVID-19 or other infections. The same can occur with MRSA, TB, and other outbreaks as people's kidneys, lungs, brains, and hearts fight off infection on top of preexisting illness. An example I've encountered numerous times is that of a person with mild asthma who, prior to COVID-19, only needed a rescue inhaler, but after COVID-19, they develop more serious asthma symptoms. Weeks or months afterward, they need a daily steroid inhaler to control symptoms, in addition to their rescue inhaler. Without looking at people's level of control for these preexisting health problems after the acute phase of the outbreak has passed, these worsening health problems will likely go undetected.

This one element of detecting a worsened preexisting condition supposes that anyone was checking in the first place. Unfortunately, providing competent chronic care is a common weakness of correctional health. The two basic areas I look at to determine whether chronic care is competent are how timely encounters are and whether the encounters are appropriate. In terms of timing, it's a long-practiced trick behind bars for correctional health systems to make an appointment for a patient then cancel it and make another. The patient may be blamed for refusing their appointment, or the appointment may simply be cancelled without telling them. In many systems, this will make the appointments appear as if they occur on time based on the days passed between the appointment being made and taking place. Even in systems with electronic medical records, it may require a laborious review of individual patient records to get at the truth of delays caused by low staffing or other systemic barriers to care. This is a central focus for people like me who investigate or monitor care, but when I start a new case, it's often apparent that the health administrators of the jail or prison don't have a transparent system to track these delays. Reporting on the Arizona prison system's problems with this issue included testimony from a mental-health counselor:

> [Her] testimony called the very nature of the medical records used by the monitoring team into question.
>
> She told the court that entries and descriptions of services provided could be backdated to make it appear they had been performed on time when they were not.
>
> [She] also provided the court with several examples of medical notes that had been written by a registered nurse but entered into the monitoring system as if they were performed by a psychiatrist.
>
> In other instances [she] said she was told what to write to ensure that her records would show up as compliant in the monitoring report.[23]

Delay or denial of these medical encounters isn't always so nuanced, however. In my work investigating the Florida prison system, patients in solitary confinement reported that correctional staff often try to bribe them with extra food or threaten them with taking away their property and clothes if they don't agree to skip medical appointments.[24] Returning to outbreaks, these types of barriers to care call into question whether people with chronic health problems are being seen frequently enough so that worsening of their asthma, diabetes, heart or kidney disease, seizures, or any other chronic problem would ever be detected in the wake of acute infection.

Another way inadequate chronic care can mask health decline after acute infection involves what happens once a patient finally gets to see a doctor or nurse practitioner for their preexisting health problem. Central to making this encounter adequate is whether the provider reviews the data about how well controlled the patient's problem is and then makes an assessment and plan based on this level of control. For example, in the asthma scenario, there are basic questions providers should ask people with asthma about how often they use their rescue inhaler, how many and how often they experience various symptoms, and how their peak-flow measurement may have changed.[25] This standard approach allows the provider to assess the level of control of the patient's asthma and decide if they need more, the same, or less treatment. The same principle applies to most chronic health problems, so that a person with high blood pressure or diabetes would have their relevant information reviewed (what they report, what the provider sees, and what labs or other tests show) to come to a similar assessment and plan.

What patients report, however, is that they get in to see a provider and are never asked these types of questions—there's a rubber-stamp approach to simply continuing everything the same way as before. These deficiencies may occur because of a lack of standardized training among providers or lack of sufficient review of their encounters by medical directors. As a result, when a person's preexisting health issue worsens after COVID-19, MRSA, or any other infection during an outbreak, it's very possible there is no reliable baseline of their illness measured beforehand.

Fortunately, a few basic interventions could make a tremendous difference in how and whether chronic problems resulting from outbreaks are detected and treated. The first and most basic move is for every facility's pandemic and infection-control plan to include an explicit mandate to track and treat these chronic problems. After an outbreak, this approach can be as simple as asking two questions of anyone who contracted the infection:

1. Does the patient have any persistent or ongoing symptoms of the infection?
2. Does the patient have any preexisting health problems that have worsened?

This type of encounter should be with a physician or mid-level provider and should happen a few weeks after the acute phase of a person's infection is thought to have finished. This allows not only for detection of untreated or partially treated infections but also for some resolution of mild symptoms to occur. When I recommend this post-outbreak encounter, correctional health administrators often tell me it isn't needed because patients already have access to care by making a sick call. When I discuss the idea with the head physician or nurse in these settings, however, they generally see the benefit both for patients and for their health service in tracking the incidence of protracted illness. But the barriers to care in jails, prisons, and immigration detention centers are largely about a lack of resources and oversight, so decisions that bring more cost and transparency are doubly resisted, even if they'd mean better patient care.

The ability of COVID-19 and other types of infections to cause prolonged or chronic health problems after so-called recovery from the acute infection is not unique to incarcerated patients. But these aspects of outbreaks receive almost no attention behind bars, despite ample evidence and guidance about how to find and treat them. One thing I've learned from correctional outbreaks is that many of the people who are initially infected are never diagnosed. As a result, symptoms that persist for weeks or months may never be attributed to the correct initial cause. This lack of attribution can lead to disability and death after the acute infection if the link is hidden. Also, the focus of correctional health services on acute care results in little identification of ongoing symptoms and illness for people who are diagnosed with infection but aren't hospitalized or gravely ill. These are two different ways an outbreak can lead to ongoing or chronic illness, but they both have the same basic fix: to incorporate persistent or chronic illness into how we respond to outbreaks behind bars.

Recommendations
- Federal and state agencies should work to add a checkbox on all death certificates to indicate whether a person died in custody, following Dr. Mitchell's recommendation.
- All carceral systems should have an independent review of deaths, with public reporting of findings and corrective action plans.
- The CDC should undertake periodic review of morbidity and mortality from outbreaks in carceral settings and make follow-up recommendations.
- Carceral settings should report on the total number and locations of people locked in a cell for 22 or more hours per day, categorizing people who have serious mental illness or acute behavioral health issues, those being punished, and those in other categories of solitary confinement.
- Infection-control staffing (including the amount of full-time equivalent workers) should be specified in contracts with for-profit vendors, and fines should be imposed for repeated or extended failures to fill these positions.

Research ideas

- Hypothesis: A significant percentage of deaths classi-
  fied as resulting from "natural causes" during outbreaks are jail- or prison-attributable; meaning, they
  were essentially caused by care or practices behind
  bars. Approach: Review deaths from a specific system
  or from public information in lawsuits to determine
  whether the medical examiner's determination of a
  "natural causes" death obscures denials of care or
  inadequate care during an outbreak.
- Hypothesis: People held in solitary confinement,
  mental-health cells, and other types of cells that are
  locked for all or most of the day experience barriers to
  adequate care during outbreaks. Approach: Review
  records of hospitalizations and deaths for overrepre-
  sentation of people in these settings. Speak with
  formerly incarcerated people and public defenders
  about access to care during outbreaks in these
  settings.
- Hypothesis: People develop unaddressed or undocumented disability and chronically worsened health
  after outbreaks. Approach: Speak with formerly
  incarcerated people and public defenders about health
  status before and after outbreaks behind bars. Review
  lawsuits that may provide information in this area.[26]

CHAPTER FOUR

The Farmville Superspreader Event

From the moment I entered the housing area, it was clear that something was wrong. I'd just arrived at Farmville Detention Center in Virginia, expecting to visit a housing area with people talking and walking around, as was usually the case in an open dorm. But here, I was surprised right away by how quiet the area was and how people were sitting at the back of the unit, arms crossed, angry. Something was going on beyond the normal stress of a COVID-19 outbreak. I headed for a large group of people and introduced myself as an outside doctor, here to find out what was happening with the COVID-19 outbreak. What they told me was a story of indifference to their health and maddening discrepancies between what immigration officials were reporting and the reality they were experiencing. The anger they shared stemmed from a series of actions by Immigration and Customs Enforcement (ICE) that would transform a facility without any COVID-19 cases into the site of one of the nation's worst superspreader events behind bars. As I focused on these core COVID-19 issues in my court-ordered inspection of the Farmville Detention Center, reporting would soon emerge tying grave errors in the facility's management of COVID-19 to a much larger effort by ICE to move their security staff around the nation in an apparent effort to put down Black Lives Matter protests in nearby Washington, DC, and circumvent rules about transferring federal law-enforcement staff. The result of those errors would be one of the most expansive COVID-19 superspreader events behind bars, with almost 90% of people in Farmville infected. Learning about the death of Mr. James Hill, as well as the way he contracted COVID-19, can help us prevent future deaths.

The timing of the Farmville superspreader event became clear during my inspection. The outbreak was triggered on June 2, 2020, when 74 people were transferred to the facility on charter flights. A total of 49 people were brought in from two ICE facilities in Arizona, and 25 came from a facility in Florida. These transfers increased the number of people in the Farmville facility from 399 to 473. When they arrived at the facility on June 2, there were no cases of COVID-19.[1] In contrast, the facilities that people were coming from—Eloy and Florence detention centers in Arizona and Krome detention center in Florida—already had many COVID-19 cases identified.[2] One of the basic recommendations made by the CDC earlier in the pandemic was to avoid transfer between detention settings because of the very predictable outcome of spreading COVID-19 from one part of the nation to another.[3] This recommendation was widely accepted by local jails and state prison systems, and even ICE had already taken steps to restrict transfers between facilities.

Like many detention settings, Farmville had set up precautions just in case new transfers into the facility did occur. In April 2020, two months before the outbreak, they established a quarantine system that required newly arrived people to spend two weeks at a nearby facility while they were monitored for COVID-19 symptoms. At the time, facilities were not yet conducting new-admission COVID-19 testing, so the best approach was to conduct daily screening for signs and symptoms and the keep newly arrived people physically separated from others for 14 days. With this system in place, Farmville could then focus on daily screening of staff as the main route of potential new infections. Over the next two months, a handful of cases were detected among newly arrived detained people, but the off-site quarantine protocol kept them isolated from the rest of the facility.

Then on the afternoon of June 1, the leadership at Farmville were notified that they would be receiving a transfer of 74 people the following day, some of whom were coming from facilities with active COVID-19 cases.[4] This number of transfers into Farmville, along with the speed and manner they were carried out, was completely unprecedented. ICE had never flown detained people from Arizona or Florida to Farmville in Virginia, and they had never transferred such a large number of detained people at one time. The sheer size of the group meant the facility's off-site quarantine unit was not big enough, so the decision was made to place all 74 people straight into Farmville. The Farmville director would state in his legal declaration that there was no indication Farmville couldn't handle this number of newly arrived people, but he also stated that "additionally, although Farmville has the right to refuse transfer of anyone whose needs cannot be accommodated at our facility, doing so here would have been impractical because we would have still been required to accept the transferees temporarily until ICE found a suitable alternative location."[5] When I met with this director, I asked about the capacity to refuse transfers for health and safety reasons, and he and his staff told me that not only could they block transfers but that they had done so in the past.[6]

Despite whatever reluctance existed, the Farmville facility was notified and then in less than 24 hours received 74 people from Arizona and Florida. And COVID-19 symptoms were evident as soon as people arrived. Two of the people from Arizona had fevers and were sent to a local hospital for COVID-19 testing before being sent into medical isolation cells at Farmville. One of their tests would come back positive and one negative on June 5. The other 72 people were placed in two open-bay dorms with bunk beds and shared bathroom facilities. Inside these tightly packed rooms, the number of people with COVID-19 symptoms would grow each day. By the middle of June, almost all the newcomers were either known to be COVID-19 positive or exhibiting symptoms. The transfer of people with suspected or known COVID-19 into single cells for medical isolation quickly became impossible based on the growing number of cases, and two dorms were used to house them. The following week, cases started to erupt among the rest of the detained people and staff at Farmville. As the outbreak grew, one of the detained people who got sick was a man named James Hill.[7]

Like so many other deaths behind bars, the death of Mr. Hill would be presented by ICE with a focus on his recent criminal incarceration, avoiding any mention of errors or deficiencies in the COVID-19 response at Farmville. Mr. Hill was 72 when he contracted COVID-19 in Farmville Detention Center, and he died less than a month later, in August 2020.[8] One of the striking things about the circumstances around his death is that his family in Canada took basic COVID-19 precautions to prepare for his arrival that

ICE did not. Having just finished a prison sentence for fraud, Mr. Hill was ordered deported to Canada, and ICE determined he should be detained for the few weeks this would take. To get ready for his arrival from the United States, where the pandemic was in full swing, his family made changes to their Toronto home so Mr. Hill could quarantine there for two weeks apart from the rest of the family.[9] This basic step—establishing a quarantine period and location—had also been identified by the CDC as an important part of preventing the spread of the virus behind bars back in March.[10] As I described above, even Farmville Detention Center had established such a protocol to house newly arrived people in a separate location and monitor them for COVID-19 symptoms before they entered the main detention center. But of course, in the weeks before Mr. Hill's death, this protocol got swept aside, and he and more than 70 other people moved directly into Farmville.

Case Study Analysis

The ICE press release reports that Mr. Hill died on August 5. He first reported symptoms of COVID-19 to Farmville staff on July 10 and was hospitalized the following day.[11] While I was unable to review Mr. Hill's medical records for my inspection, if I had been able to see them, I would have focused on when he'd first experienced symptoms versus when he'd received care. During my inspection, I asked 20 detained people about sick call—a process used by people in detention to report illness or a new medical problem. The facility had told me that anyone reporting serious health problems, including COVID-19 symptoms, would be seen within 24 hours if not sooner. As I wrote in my report, of the 20 detained people I spoke with, "14 of them reported personally submitting sick call requests, 10 of them for COVID-19-related symptoms, and not one of them reported being seen within 24 hours."[12] When I asked facility leadership whether adherence to this policy was tracked, I was told there was no such quality-assurance monitoring but that compliance was "100%."[13] This disconnect—between the deficiencies reported by patients and the accounts by staff of total compliance—would be reconcilable in other settings like community health systems, where this type of crucial process would be monitored by quality assurance to determine not only the timing of encounters but also whether they were adequately preformed. But by failing to track this process, the Farmville Detention Center (and many other correctional health services) forced conflict between the official version of events and the reports of patients who actually receive care. In the context of detention settings with vast power imbalances between the patients and the staff, this lack of verification can give outsiders the false impression that things are fine. Simply accepting the facility leadership's version of events when they offer a glowing self-assessment such as something happening correctly "100%" of the time also promotes the assumption that detained people are not credible, which can discourage them from reporting problems as they expect a lack of response. Often during my inspections, people who have spent more time in a facility will report they simply gave up on parts of the health service that don't work. I've often heard from people I interview that the costs of continuing to submit sick-call requests and grievances, in both financial and retaliation terms, can quickly outweigh the benefits when care is delayed or nonexistent.

Often the response to reports of delayed sick calls places the blame on patients, either for being untrustworthy, or for not following the rules or procedures. For example, the medical expert hired by ICE in the Farmville case stated in his report, "The Detainees are generally unhappy with their detention, and each has a list of complaints. The first is with regard to time to being seen at sick call. There is an extensive education process imparted to the Detainees regarding procedure for putting in a sick call request. The Detainees are issued a booklet of these procedures, are shown a video, and have personal education from medical staff. Interpretation services ensure that there is no language barrier. Failure to follow proper procedure can result in a delay in being seen at sick call."[14]

While it is true that not understanding the rules of the sick-call process could result in delays, the focus on this as the main or sole cause of deficiencies, and the lack of any system to monitor the adherence of the facility in terms of their staffing or ability to deliver on their obligations, is characteristic of historical correctional-health standard practices: blame the patient and don't measure whether the care is adequate or timely. This is an area where many detention settings have improved, especially with the introduction of electronic medical records (EMR). In most of the facilities with EMR, it is relatively easy to measure the sick-call response time, both for the initial review by a nurse as well as the face-to-face encounter.

An even more glaring disconnect existed at Farmville over the failure to address (or even acknowledge) the actual cause of the outbreak. Anger swelled among detained people about ICE causing the outbreak with the transfer of so many un-quarantined people because only *after* causing this calamity did ICE and Farmville get serious about infection control by mandating masks and having the CDC perform testing. The

CDC deployed a team to Farmville shortly before I was there, and their report includes meticulous detail about the activities of their team and recommendations about testing, but it offers almost nothing on the root causes of the outbreak. The report provides results of additional testing the team conducted, a timeline of events up to their visit, and a discussion of staff surveys. But despite having spent an extensive amount of time inside the facility, it's unclear whether CDC staff learned from detained people themselves.[15] For example, in my inspection, I asked 21 people whether the daily COVID-19 screenings that occur during quarantine involve temperature checks *and* asking about COVID-19 symptoms. The facility leadership told me both temperature checks *and* specific symptom questions occur for every person every day they are screened in quarantine.[16] The CDC report states without any qualification, "Currently, all detained persons are screened for fever and COVID-19-like symptoms at least once per day and have the opportunity to be screened and interact with medical staff twice a day during 'pill call.'"[17] But among the 21 people I asked about this process, 19 stated that no such symptom questions were asked of them, and 2 said that occasionally general wellness questions were asked. People also reported that no interpreter was used during these screenings.[18] The CDC team appeared to take their impression of what occurs in this process directly from the leadership of the facility, not the people detained there. By simply accepting this version of events, the CDC team placed a heavy stamp of approval on the facility's response, notably accepting that new instances of COVID-19 symptoms were being effectively detected. The facility director also told the Farmville town council in August 2020 that nobody in the facility had experienced a single symptom of COVID-19 since July 10, an assurance at odds with statements from detained people but one the CDC report falls squarely in line with.[19]

In my inspection, I also learned that about half the detained people were Spanish speaking but most health staff were not.[20] To make matters worse, the conclusion section of the CDC report on Farmville begins, "The COVID-19 outbreak in the FDC was difficult to manage and mitigate due to the housing design and limited number of rooms to medically isolate or quarantine persons who were sick or were waiting for test results to return."[21] Not a single finding or conclusion is offered about the way the outbreak was caused by the transfer of people from facilities with active outbreaks, or about the fact that the spread of infection and the death of Mr. Hill were avoidable and were the direct result of putting aside existing quarantine measures. This lack of accountability is common in correctional settings, but this report was especially depressing to read because the hope in involving the CDC in measuring and promoting health among detained people has always been to bring transparency and accountability about the health risks of incarceration. The mission of the CDC is to protect public health, but reading this report, it was difficult to see how ignoring the obvious root cause of the outbreak represented protecting the public health of detained people.

The outbreak at Farmville is a classic superspreader event, but we mustn't conclude that it was an unavoidable tragedy. There are several definitions of the term "superspreader," but they all involve a small number of index cases causing infection in a much larger number. One well-documented example of a superspreader event is a scientific conference in Boston, Massachusetts, in which 90 COVID-19 cases among conference participants led to thousands of other cases as the infected participants traveled home.[22] But the conference in Boston occurred in February 2020, before the threat from COVID-19 was generally known and certainly before there were guidelines about how to prevent and manage this pandemic. The superspreader event at Farmville happened in June 2020, many months after guidelines were provided by the CDC on how to quarantine newly arrived people and avoid inter-facility spread. But as we've seen, ICE and Farmville set aside their own protocols and took unprecedented logistical steps to make this transfer in a hasty manner.

The reasons for the massive transfer of people and why the seemingly effective quarantine protocols were swept aside eluded me during my inspection, and nobody, including the director of the facility, would offer any explanations. A couple of weeks after I left Farmville, investigative reporting from Antonio Olivo and Nick Miroff at the *Washington Post* revealed a part of this story that was beyond my wildest imagination. Basically, they found that detained people were moved to help hide and justify the movement of federal agents, not for any ICE reasons. The first sentence of their bombshell story reads, "The Trump administration flew immigrant detainees to Virginia this summer to facilitate the rapid deployment of Homeland Security tactical teams to quell protests in Washington, circumventing restrictions on the use of charter flights for employee travel, according to a current and a former US official."[23] The details of the reporting focus on a prohibition against ICE agents flying on charter flights unless detainees were also on board. The transfer of detainees from multiple parts of the country to the Washington, DC, area would apparently allow ICE to move their special-response-team agents without running afoul of this regulation. The article supports this allegation with multiple sources, and cites an ICE lawyer who told a judge the transfer was in part necessitated because "ICE has an air regulation whereby in order to move agents of ICE, they have to be moved from one location to another with detainees on the same airplane."[24] So, what did these special-response agents do once in DC? A leaked memo from the Trump administration lays out how over 1,500 federal law-enforcement workers were deployed to quell Black Lives Matter and other protests that were occurring in response to the killing of George Floyd. This memo mentions approximately 700 agents were from the Department of Homeland Security, including ICE officers.[25] Publicly, ICE made the incredible claim that these transfers were part of a COVID-19 mitigation plan. The director of ICE enforcement stated, "The June 2 transfer of detainees to Farmville was made as part of a national effort to spread detainees across the detention network to facilitate social distancing and mitigate the spread of COVID-19."[26] But the *Washington Post* reporting also makes clear that the sending facilities were not at or near capacity,[27] and both common sense and CDC guidelines at the time make the director's claim not credible.

The folly of the move was apparent well before it occurred, even inside ICE and Farmville. The *Washington Post* piece refers to an August meeting of the Farmville town council. In the video of this meeting, the director of Farmville Detention Center states he had already made a recommendation to ICE before June not to transfer more detained people into the facility, which was ignored. He also states the local ICE field office "pushed back" and attempted to block the June 2 transfer into Farmville, but officials in Washington, DC, overrode the objections. He adds that an assurance he received from ICE about detained people coming from facilities not having COVID-19 wasn't accurate. He responds to a question about the apparent moratorium on transfers in the ICE system by stating, "The fallout for ICE as a result of the June 2 transfers has caused the great consternation, as it should."[28] No questions in this meeting focused on the facility putting aside its preexisting new-admission quarantine.

Farmville itself has a long history of sitting at the crossroads of struggles for civil rights—and local governments have been on all sides. I didn't know until my inspection, but Farmville students played a pivotal role in the *Brown v. Board of Education* decision by the US Supreme Court regarding school desegregation. In the early 1950s, students and their parents led a school walkout protesting conditions and resources in the local high school for Black students. This case would be combined with several others in the Supreme Court's landmark decision in 1954, but the response of the county (Prince Edward) was not to comply but to close the school altogether. This resistance to desegregation was voted on locally and was part of a statewide program to maintain school segregation well into the 1960s. As a result, many local teachers lost their jobs, and many African American students went without a formal high-school education, earning the term the "lockout generation." Decades later, residents would protest the start of the ICE presence in Farmville, and they would continue protesting up to and following the death of James Hill.

The modern relationship between the town of Farmville and the detention center is a complex one. Importantly, the detention center provides jobs in a rural setting where they are scarce, and the town itself also reaps direct financial benefits from the facility. The National Immigrant Justice Center conducted a review of the financial ties between the company Immigration Centers of America Inc. and the town of Farmville. The review shows the town is not only rewarded financially through the presence of the detention center, but it acts as the intermediary between ICE and the company, so that ICE contracts with the town, which in turn contracts with the company. The total financial compensation is reduced to a per diem or per head payment for holding detained people, which started as $79.89 in 2008 and has climbed to $120.75. This complicated arrangement doesn't stop ICE from negotiating directly with the company, but it keeps the town involved as an ally, as a recipient of some share of the revenue, and as a paymaster, with ICE sending funds to the town, which sends them on to the company.[29] The inspector general of the Department of Homeland Security has been critical of convoluted financial arrangements between ICE and for-profit detention centers, but deals like the one with Farmville remain common.[30] So, this financial relationship creates a partnership between the town, the company Immigration Centers of America Inc., and ICE, based on the business of detaining immigrants. What the superspreader event and death of Mr. Hill reveal is that this partnership is not one that requires the town of Farmville to step in when the facility's recommendations are overruled or to demand accountability when an outbreak occurs.

Examples of What Works

James Hill's death and the Farmville superspreader event must be considered as preventable and the outcome of human errors. The detention center had a process in place to quarantine newly arrived people off site, and this process appeared to be working, with only sporadic cases appearing before June 2. The events that transpired starting June 2, leading to the death of Mr. Hill and the infection of most of the other people in the facility, are not really in question. The lack of accountability for causing this outbreak, however, is not only a problem within ICE but also extends to the CDC, which came, inspected, and conducted surveys and testing but failed to comment on the obvious cause of the outbreak and death. Another concern raised by this event should be the ease with which ICE was able to steamroll the for-profit company into accepting detained people over multiple levels of objections. Most correctional settings can refuse transfers in of people who pose a public-health risk or who are not medically cleared.

The town of Farmville should have played an important role in stopping these transfers, but it did not. And the company, Immigration Centers of America Inc., does not appear to have raised their concerns outside their internal discussions with ICE. Taken together, all these actors displayed a shocking disregard for the welfare of the people detained by ICE and the obvious worsening of the pandemic they would contribute to. The position later taken by ICE, that the transfers were some sort of public-health response to COVID-19, is a final and incredible bit of hypocrisy. The problems revealed by this case are deep and systemic inside the ICE detention system, and inside the CDC, which was able to become involved in a public-health catastrophe and remain silent on the causes.

These failures at Farmville gave rise to the seething hostility that develops among people when their captors tell the outside world a version of events they know to be untrue. I wrote in my Farmville report that "the level of animosity and disengagement among detainees is more acute at FDC than any other facility I have inspected, and flows directly from the reality that widespread COVID-19 was caused by the mass transfers into the facility in June and that the predictable consequences of these transfers, detainees becoming ill, were ignored by staff."[31] The path forward must involve challenging the ICE detention system but also a more rigorous and reliable role by the CDC, as well as local and state health agencies. Such changes will require the political will to prioritize health outcomes among immigrants and people of color as worthy of attention, effort, and protection.

Recommendations

- Independent, expert review of ICE health services is needed. This should include annual reporting based on unannounced inspections and medical-records reviews by outside experts to assess ICE compliance with their own policies on general health services and with CDC recommendations during outbreaks.[32]
- Detention of people with serious medical or behavioral health problems should be reconsidered, especially when active outbreaks are underway and when resources for health services are not available.
- Local and state relationships with ICE that involve payment for detention of undocumented immigrants in for-profit detention centers need much more scrutiny from health departments.
- When the CDC reviews or investigates an outbreak in a detention setting, their findings should include and publicly report on contributing causes and corrective action plans.

- EMR implementation should include a basic set of quality measures, including sick-call timeliness and adequacy.

Research ideas

- Hypothesis: ICE assessments of the adequacy of care they provide lack important elements used by local organizations such as state departments of health and federal Medicare and Medicaid standards, and may even lack basic elements used by the US Bureau of Prisons to review care. Approach: Review internal ICE facility audits and Department of Homeland Security Office of Inspector General (OIG) assessments for content on outbreaks and infections.[33] Compare the methods of these reports to state health departments, federal Medicare and Medicaid, as well as Bureau of Prison audits and those from the Joint Commission.
- Hypothesis: Infection-control staffing in ICE facilities may be deficient. Approach: Review OIG and other reports on ICE health-care staffing, including infection-control staff. Review lawsuits that may provide information in this area.[34]

CHAPTER FIVE

Heat

W elcome to hell." That's the greeting 58-year-old Larry Gene McCollum got when he arrived at the Hutchins State Jail in Texas to serve a 12-month sentence for forgery.[1] He showed up during an especially hot July in 2011, and a few days later, he died from the heat. Like most Texas prisons, Hutchins didn't have full air-conditioning coverage, and the temperatures inside and outside rose well beyond 90°F, with a far higher heat index.[2] When he arrived, Mr. McCollum had two medical issues that made him heat sensitive, meaning that each of these conditions increased his risk of heat-related illness and death. He was morbidly obese with a body mass index of 49, and he had hypertension. When he first got to Hutchins, his family reports there was some distribution of water, but he couldn't buy his own cup to drink water, and he couldn't buy a fan. Also, his initial medical screening, which wasn't with a physician, resulted in his blood-pressure medicine being switched from clonidine to hydrochlorothi-azide. This is relevant because the new medication was a diuretic, which can cause dehydration and is known to increase risk from heat stress. In addition, Mr. McCollum wasn't scheduled to get his intake physical with a doctor until a week after his arrival, so in those initial days of incarceration, he didn't receive any heat-sensitivity protections like work restrictions, special housing, or a bottom bunk despite his morbid obesity, hypertension, and being prescribed a diuretic.

Mr. McCollum was sent to a dorm where the windows were sealed shut and where 57 other men were housed. He initially found a bottom bunk but was forced to move to a top one the following day because someone else had a medical order for a bottom bunk. The lawsuit filed by his family reports that he became unable to get up and down from the bunk, so he stopped going to meals, and other people in his dorm grew worried about his health within a few days. About a week into his stay, another incarcerated person reported to a correctional officer that Mr. McCollum was shaking. The officer who observed Mr. McCollum also saw him in convulsions. After an hour of phone calls to various supervisors and off-site staff, 911 was eventually called. By this time, Mr. McCollum's apparent seizures had stopped. Because of his size, five EMTs were required to remove Mr. McCollum from his top bunk and transport him to nearby Parkland Memorial Hospital.

When he arrived, Mr. McCollum's body temperature was 109.4°F. He died shortly afterward, and the autopsy report identified the cause of death as "the result of hyperthermia. The decedent was in a hot environment without air conditioning, and he may have been further predisposed to developing hyperthermia due to morbid obesity and treatment with a diuretic for hypertension."[3] Mr. McCollum was one of 11 people to die from heat-related illness during the summer of 2011 in the Texas prisons.[4]

Case Study Analysis

The rapid pace of deaths from heat-related illness in Texas prisons in 2011, including Mr. McCollum's death, meets the CDC definition of an outbreak: "an increase of disease among a specific population in a geographic area during a specific period of time."[5] In this case, the outbreak was driven by the extreme weather, lack of air-conditioning, and the personal risk factors of the people who died.

Outbreaks can originate from infection passing from one person to another, like influenza, MRSA, and scabies. But outbreaks can also be caused by rapid or unanticipated increases in other diseases, like illnesses from contaminated food or water, and even illnesses triggered by environmental factors like heat. When these outbreaks occur in jails, prisons, and detention centers, the intersection between the personal health characteristics of people and the environmental risks posed by the facility can drive rapid escalation of illness and death.

Texas has been described as ground zero for heat-related mortality behind bars because of the refusal of the prison system and state government to install air-conditioning and the terrifying number of people who have died (and continue to die) from heat-related illness in these facilities. The summer of Mr. McCollum's death had been preceded by another series of five heat-related deaths in 1998.[6]

As with most other sources of death and illness behind bars, the CDC and state department of health are essentially absent from these policy discussions, leaving families and those who want to prevent these deaths to pursue litigation. Numerous lawsuits have been filed in Texas regarding heat-related deaths. The most successful involved a single Texas prison that housed vulnerable patients, including both those with serious medical problems and the elderly. This facility, the Pack Unit, was not air-conditioned despite the concentration of heat-sensitive and frail people. After years of fierce opposition by the Texas prison system and a scathing rebuke by a federal court, a settlement was reached in 2018 that mandated air-conditioning.[7] As with many wins for the health of incarcerated people, this was not only limited in scope but met with ongoing resistance by the prison system. The settlement covered one facility, and approximately 75% of the housing areas in the rest of the 130 or so prisons were left without air-conditioning. In addition, within a year, the judge cited the prison system for failing to do what it had agreed to in the settlement. In fact, the judge became so irate with the Texas prison officials that he threatened to lock them in the same un-air-conditioned cells they so often touted as humane and acceptable. He fumed, "Shouldn't we have as a sanction, prison officials in the cells dealing with the same temperatures as the prisoners?"[8]

Ultimately, the Pack Unit got air-conditioning, but the rest of the prison system was left mostly untouched, and periodic bills to fund air-conditioning in the prisons would clear one part of state government only to be swatted down by another.[9] In late 2023, progress was finally made to significantly expand air-conditioning coverage.[10] The struggles to simply prevent deaths from heat in Texas prisons is heartbreaking for many reasons, not the least of which is the lack of leadership by the groups charged with protecting public health, the Texas Department of State Health Services and the CDC. In the past 20 years, the CDC has developed sophisticated tracking methods for heat-related illness, tallying high-heat days and numerous other aspects.[11] But their tracking tools and outbreak investigations include virtually nothing about how often people die from heat-related illness behind bars or about how these facilities should identify and protect heat-sensitive people, such as by installing air-conditioning.

As with other aspects of health behind bars, when the CDC and state departments of health are absent, litigation and local reporting provide some of the only means to establish the truth of what is happening. For example, in Texas, many of the investigations into heat-related deaths have been done by local reporters, including *Texas Tribune* reporter Jolie Mc-Cullough. Reviewing these numerous articles shows how expert investigation and reporting can reveal the health risks of incarceration in a way everyone can appreciate.[12] Unfortunately, while these approaches are critical to raise awareness, they're usually not sufficient to make widespread and lasting changes.

Families of people who have died from heat-related illness in this system have filed numerous lawsuits, some individual and some class action. Teams of attorneys have pursued this issue for decades alongside these families, but in this adversarial context, the State of Texas has pushed back on even the most elemental details. In Mr. McCollum's case, the prison's medical provider, the University of Texas Medical Branch (UTMB), disputed whether Mr. McCollum had actually taken all the doses of the diuretic he'd been prescribed when he'd arrived at Hutchins. This argument ignores the fact they judged him ill enough to need this medicine but provided no heat-related accommodations or bottom-bunk order for him. UTMB made the point in their legal filings that their records didn't show Mr. McCollum had gone to the pill window to get his medications. But the court cited the plaintiff's report that "the same records allegedly indicating that McCollum did not take his medicine also seem to indicate that McCollum took the medicine on August 8, August 12, August 13, and August 14—weeks after his death."[13] The Texas prison system also made the point in this and other cases that there was *some* air-conditioning in many of their prisons. Again, the court in Mr. McCollum's case had an astute take on this: "The majority of these prisons do not have air-conditioning in the inmate housing areas (*Id.* at 11), but all of the prisons have some areas that are air-conditioned. For example, all of the wardens' offices are air-conditioned, as are all of the regional directors' offices and the correctional officers' stations (known as 'pickets')."[14]

In other cases, the State of Texas simply stated they didn't believe a person had died from heat-related illness, despite clear evidence to the contrary and even when the autopsy identified heat as the culprit.[15] In the case of Mr. McCollum, much of the public information is from the judge's order denying the state's efforts to simply have the case dismissed or grant immunity to prison officials. The judge wrote in his order that "Larry McCollum's tragic death was not simply bad luck, but an entirely preventable consequence of inadequate policies. These policies contributed to the deaths of eleven men before McCollum and ten men after him."[16]

Even without the leadership of our public-health agencies in preventing and reporting on heat-related illness and deaths, individuals working in medicine and public health have effectively raised the alarm about heat-related illness behind bars. One of the true giants in these efforts is a friend and mentor of mine, Dr. Susi Vassallo. Dr. Vassallo is a professor of emergency medicine at NYU School of Medicine, and her work on heat sensitivity in prisons and jails ranges from the New York City jails to prisons in Louisiana, Mississippi, and Texas. In reviewing information for this chapter, I reread reports of hers spanning from 2002 in Mississippi to 2023 in Louisiana.[17] Dr. Vassallo was the medical expert in numerous other heat-illness cases, including in New York City jails, where her work with plaintiffs suing the city led to the mandate that the jail health service I joined after fellowship training screen all our patients for heat sensitivity during high-heat months. This is such a valuable tool that since learning about it while running the New York City jail health service, I have recommended it in many other places—and it comes straight from Dr. Vassallo's involvement in a case almost 20 years ago.[18]

In addition to individual case work, important developments from public-health researchers have called attention to heat-related illness behind bars. In 2022, an analysis led by Dr. Julianne Skarha and a team of seasoned epidemiologists attributed 271 deaths in Texas prisons between 2001 and 2019 to excessive heat.[19] It's worth noting the Texas prison system has said they had 0 heat-related deaths after 2012.[20] In their study, Dr. Skarha and her colleagues compared death rates in settings with and without air-conditioning, and analyzed risk factors associated with heat sensitivity. They found that "a 1-degree increase above 85°F in prisons without air conditioning was associated with a 0.7% increase in the risk of daily mortality. Approximately 13% of deaths in Texas prisons during warm months between 2001 and 2019 may be attributable to extreme heat days."[21] This work, alongside advocacy from families of incarcerated people in Texas and other states, helped force a more national discussion of the problem in 2023.[22]

Examples of What Works

As climate change brings more high-heat days to midwestern and northern states, these heat-related problems are appearing in prisons that have never had to contend with them before. Facilities outside the Deep South and Southwest have rarely needed to consider the potential for outbreaks of heat-related illness, but now it's becoming a universal concern.[23] When New Jersey's new prison ombudsman issued his first report, he chose this topic, explaining how people behind bars are especially vulnerable because of the widespread heat sensitivity among incarcerated people and the lack of air-conditioning in the state's prisons.[24] I was in the Walla Walla State Penitentiary in Washington in the summer of 2021 when the temperature during a heat wave reached 116°F. That facility happened to be mostly air-conditioned, but many people incarcerated around the state weren't in air-conditioned cells.[25] The need to identify and protect heat-sensitive people isn't limited to facilities without air-conditioning. Incarcerated people may sleep in an air-conditioned place but work in one that isn't, or vice versa. Jobs that involve working in kitchens and factories, or doing outdoor groundskeeping, all may routinely expose people to temperatures above 100°F and heat-index readings in the "danger" and "extreme-danger" zones.

Occupational exposure to heat is further complicated by the practice of forced labor behind bars. Because the 13th Amendment to the US Constitution eliminated slavery with an exception for prison labor, many incarcerated people are forced to work. Complaining about their health status can bring punishment or loss of early release opportunities.[26] Fold in the lack of Occupational Safety and Health Administration (OSHA) rules applying to prisons, and this creates a situation where forced labor is implemented however prison guards and administrators see fit.[27] OSHA has a good list of factors that increase heat sensitivity as well as guidelines to avoid heat-related illness in work settings, but these common-sense practices simply don't apply to incarcerated workers.[28] The combination of forcing people to work and failing to create transparent or accountable standards for work conditions not only harms their health, but it also makes health staff one of the only possible sources of help when a person is harmed by their work conditions. The very mandate for prison health care came from a US Supreme Court case (*Estelle v. Gamble*) in which an imprisoned man was forced back to work after a work-related back injury without intervention from medical staff.[29] This dynamic continues today, with untracked injury and illness relating to prison labor and little accountability—even when a person dies while working.

Another serious concern is the simple reality that air conditioners break, and repairs may be delayed weeks or months. When the judge in the Pack Unit threatened Texas prison officials with being locked in the same hot cells incarcerated people were experiencing, one of the reasons he found these officials had "behaved dishonorably" included their failure to fix broken or malfunctioning air-conditioning units.[30] Part of my work as a federal prison monitor has been to find and report on instances of broken air conditioners, and determine whether the heat rises to unacceptable levels and whether heat-sensitive people are protected while repairs are made. In one recent case, I received reports about a broken air conditioner, went to the facility to inspect the housing area, and was able to get temperature readings from the high-heat days when the unit was under repair. In this case, the temperatures never exceeded 85°F, and the facility also had a good handle on who was heat sensitive and implemented extra surveillance for heat-related illness. But a broken air conditioner can often lead to partial or total loss of cooling in a housing area. Because housing units are often tightly sealed when air-conditioning is first installed, temperatures can quickly soar without air-conditioning, especially in solitary-confinement cells where solid doors and a lack of windows can literally turn a cell into an oven. A heat-sensitive patient died at Rikers in 2014 when the ventilation to his cell malfunctioned, leading the cell temperature to rise to 101°F and causing him to die of heat-related illness.[31] This man, Jerome Murdough, was in a mental-health unit, and the problem with his cell's malfunctioning ventilation system was apparently known to security staff and awaiting repair. The situation was made worse because the assigned officer was off the housing area and didn't make the required rounds while Mr. Murdough became ill.[32] When Mr. Murdough was eventually discovered slumped on the floor in a pool of his blood and vomit, his cell temperature was 101°F and his internal body temperature 103°F.[33] As this case shows, delays in getting the necessary air-conditioner parts or technicians can easily go from days to weeks, and the more remote or hidden from outside eyes the facility is, the more likely it is that health problems will stay undiscovered.

There are plenty of other kinds of outbreaks behind bars not caused by communicable diseases or person-to-person transmission, including outbreaks of foodborne illness and poisoning from environmental toxins like lead and arsenic. One of the more common examples is a salmonella outbreak, like the one in 2011 in the Canaan federal prison in

Pennsylvania that sickened over 300 people.[34] Another outbreak from 2012 in Arkansas state prisons sickened over 500 people at two facilities. The culprit was initially identified as a potato salad.[35] But when the CDC investigated, they detected eight different serotypes of salmonella in the stool samples of incarcerated people. Their investigation concluded that multiple levels of failure occurred, which led to salmonella-contaminated eggs being provided to the facilities, problems with food storage and preparation, and inadequate training for the incarcerated people who worked in these roles. The CDC also identified at least some person-to-person transmission in this case, showing how people in remote prisons with inadequate agricultural- and food-safety practices can suffer a complex outbreak.[36] In 2017, the CDC offered their first review of foodborne illness in correctional settings in 20 years, and they found that 200 outbreaks occurred, causing over 20,000 illnesses, 204 hospitalizations, and 5 deaths. They also reported that the most common causes of these outbreaks were the bacteria salmonella and clostridium, as well as norovirus. The most common contributing factor in the outbreaks was food remaining at room temperature. Finally, the CDC established that illness from foodborne outbreaks behind bars represented 6% of all cases in the nation and that the rate of illness from these outbreaks was almost seven times higher behind bars than in the community.[37]

We can see how this type of unchecked infection and lack of basic prevention and detection measures for prison workers is especially dangerous when we consider cases of people in the United States with bird flu (H5N1, or avian influenza). The most recent case involved a farmworker who'd had contact with infected cattle in Texas in 2023; the case before that was a person who'd worked with poultry in Colorado in 2022.

Both people had relatively mild symptoms and recovered.[38] For decades, these kinds of sporadic cases have happened around the world. But a new US development is the presence of widespread infection across millions of birds and farm animals in multiple states. This increases the risk of animal-to-human transmission as well as the more dangerous prospect that mutations will eventually lead to human-to-human transmission. This concern is relevant to prison outbreaks because of the widespread reliance on incarcerated people to work in many types of farming and food preparation.[39]

Water contamination with lead and arsenic has also been identified as a potential cause of outbreaks in prison and jail settings.[40] Because prison and jail water sources and filtration and purification systems are often similar to those in the local community, there is an overlap between poorly protected water sources in rural and low-income areas with the problems faced by nearby prison and jails.[41] One relatively rare type of outbreak behind bars involves botulism poisoning from making hooch or pruno, a homemade wine common behind bars. Pruno is made by fermenting everyday food items, but when the bacteria *Clostridium botulinum* is present, it can produce a deadly toxin that causes nerve damage and sometimes respiratory paralysis. This type of illness has been reported to the CDC from jails and prisons in multiple states, including California, Utah, Mississippi, and Arizona.[42] In the Mississippi outbreak, the symptoms were mostly mild, such as cranial nerve problems like dry mouth, hoarse voice, and difficulty swallowing, along with fatigue and abdominal cramps.[43] The worry is that a larger dose of the bacterial toxin could lead to paralysis and difficulty breathing.

***

These types of outbreaks pose significant threats to the lives of incarcerated people (and staff), but there is one key distinction between heat-related illnesses and the salmonella, clostridium, arsenic, lead, and even botulism outbreaks. The latter are all types of infections or toxicity reported to state and federal health and environmental agencies—and for which there are standardized methods to investigate, track, and report illness. For heat, on the other hand, there are no standards about how to prevent, identify, and respond to related illness behind bars. In Texas, the governor recently signed a bill to eliminate a state law mandating water breaks for construction workers. Texas had the most heat-related occupational deaths *before* this bill was signed.[44] For incarcerated workers who also lack even the most basic OSHA protections, this signals more disregard for their survival in high-heat conditions. Taken together, the information we have today shows that heat-related illness is a hidden, deadly, and expanding threat to health behind bars.

There are clear best practices for investigations into heat-related outbreaks. One of the most memorable moments proving this fact for me came in the 1990s when a heat wave in the Midwest led to hundreds of deaths in Chicago, mostly among poor people and people of color living in public housing. The CDC conducted a rigorous investigation and published a *Morbidity and Mortality Weekly Report* on this rolling tragedy of heat-related deaths. One of the core assessments from this 1995 report remains both true and unaddressed behind bars: "Heat-related mortality is preventable. The most effective measures for preventing heat-related illness and death include reducing physical activity, drinking additional nonalcoholic liquids, and increasing the amount of time spent in air-conditioned environments."[45]

Recommendations

Outbreaks of heat-related illness are predicable, considering we know that all jails, prisons, and detention centers have a significant share of heat-sensitive people in their custody and that many or most of these facilities will contend with temperatures that exceed 85°F at some time. Despite knowing who is heat sensitive, most carceral facilities have yet to adopt a standardized approach to keeping track of this vulnerable cohort, including monitoring where they live and work.

- Support state and federal laws that eliminate forced labor, protect incarcerated workers from heat and other harmful conditions, and mandate fair wages.
- Mandate identification and clinical surveillance of all heat-sensitive incarcerated people as well as staff whenever temperatures exceed 85°F, ensuring their living, transportation, and work settings are air-conditioned.
- To the CDC: replicate your reviews of foodborne illness, COVID-19, and other outbreaks in carceral settings for heat-related illness. Provide basic recommendations on preventing and responding to heat-related illness.

Research ideas

- Hypothesis: Rates of heat-related death increase during high-heat periods in jails and prisons. Approach: Replicate Dr. Skarha's approach in other settings and match heat-mortality data to incarceration data, as was similarly done to match fatal-overdose data to incarceration data to establish post-release overdose increases.[46] Review lawsuits that may provide information in this area.[47]

- Hypothesis: Lax rules and oversight of work conditions in prisons can contribute to outbreaks. Approach: Examine outbreaks with food or agricultural elements to determine whether or how a lower standard of hygiene and infection control may have contributed to the outbreak. As part of this examination, review contracts that involve incarcerated people being "loaned out" to businesses and consider how their conditions may differ from nonincarcerated employees.[48]

CHAPTER SIX

The Incredible Itch

Scabies Outbreaks

Wendy Snead was almost done with a five-month sentence in a Tennessee prison when a woman with a head-to-toe rash was transferred into her eight-person pod from another one in the facility. Although the newly arrived woman said she wasn't contagious, one woman in their housing area had had nursing training and expressed worry that the rash was from scabies. The women already living in the pod complained to staff about the arrival of someone with an obvious rash, and they even refused to be housed near her. It turned out the newly arrived woman had already endured several months of trying to get medical staff to pay attention to her ailment. She had filed numerous grievances and made repeated efforts to get help with the painful, itching rash. Soon, not surprisingly, the women in Ms. Snead's pod started to experience similar symptoms themselves, and they discussed these symptoms as a scabies outbreak. Instead of sending medical staff in to track the spread of cases, and to screen and care for the women, facility guards threatened the detained women with solitary confinement if they further discussed any scabies outbreak.

During this time, Ms. Snead noticed several itchy and painful red bumps on her right arm. This was almost five months after the woman with the original rash had first tried and failed to receive treatment. Ms. Snead showed her rash to a nurse, who told Ms. Snead to change the soap she was using, despite her having used the same institutional soap without any problems during the previous four months of her incarceration.[1]

Scabies is an infection and infestation caused by a tiny parasite called a "mite." When pregnant female mites find their way onto human skin, they burrow into the outer layers and lay a few eggs a day.[2] The mites themselves aren't usually visible to the naked eye, but the burrowing and egg laying causes raised red or purple lines on the skin. This also causes extreme itching, especially at night. One of the unique things about scabies is that the first signs of infection take weeks to show in people who have never been infected before, but most people with prior infection mount a rapid allergy and inflammatory response that results in symptoms within days. Both groups can easily pass the mites to others for the entire time they have the parasites on their skin. As a result, scabies outbreaks are common in closely packed settings like day cares, schools, and detention facilities. Having scabies is often referred to as an "infestation" as opposed to an "infection," since the parasites remain outside the body.[3] Treatment for scabies involves applying a prescribed cream or lotion to the skin, but outbreak response also requires knowing how extensive the cases are, washing clothes and linens effectively, and keeping infected people away from others.

One reason scabies outbreaks are ignored is that most people experience maddening itching and skin lesions but don't require hospitalization or become seriously ill. But for people with compromised immune systems, instead of being infected with 10–15 mites, their skin may be colonized by thousands or even millions of mites, and they can face life-threatening secondary infections that enter their blood-stream. If someone isn't aware of a scabies infestation, or they're ignored in an isolated space, scabies can cover their entire body and, again, become life-threatening. This was the case for a 93-year-old nursing-home patient in Georgia who died from what an autopsy report characterized as "septice-mia encrusted scabies."[4] A forensic pathologist involved in the case estimated that hundreds of millions of mites likely in-fested this patient's body over months to years.[5] This horrible case is relevant for scabies behind bars because, like many other health risks of incarceration, severe scabies infestations are more likely to occur among people with serious mental ill-ness who are locked away in a cell and essentially left there for weeks, months, or years with minimal assessment of their physical health.

Ms. Snead submitted additional sick-call requests for care but was ignored, which led her to submit several grievances about the lack of care and even a direct complaint to the fa-cility's assistant warden. As a result of her complaints, she was placed in lockdown, preventing her from having contact with her family. Eventually, Ms. Snead was given an appointment with a dermatologist outside the facility, who promptly diag-nosed scabies and prescribed treatments, which the facility then refused to obtain for her. She was also placed back into lockdown after her return from the appointment, again out of contact with others. Days later, Ms. Snead was released at the end of her sentence. Still suffering from scabies, she finally received definitive care at an emergency department, but she also incurred considerable costs to clean her home and pay for medications. When she shared her experience in the facility with her family, they reported her concerns to the Nashville department of health. Two letters signed by dozens of women would also make their way to the health department, reporting the outbreak and lack of treatment. The woman who'd originally reported scabies symptoms in this case would tell a judge during a hearing that she was unable to go to her court-ordered prison program after release because of her untreated scabies, which she'd reported and sought treatment for in the facility for almost five months. Throughout the 1,300-bed facility, hundreds of other women had to be treated for scabies during this outbreak, although there was virtually no monitoring or record of the problems they encountered in getting treatment inside the facility or when they returned home. Multiple lawsuits would be filed by women held at the facility during the scabies outbreak, leading to a class-action suit and eventually to at least $150,000 in financial settlements paid by CoreCivic, the private prison company running the facility, to Ms. Snead and the other women who experienced scabies and denials of care.[6]

Case Study Analysis

If scabies or another outbreak occurred in a Nashville nursing home, or school, facility staff would likely report the problem right away to department of health experts, triggering contact tracing, efforts to determine the scope of the problem and the best way to prevent further spread, and efforts to provide treatment. When the scabies outbreak happened in CoreCivic's private prison, it was the patients themselves and their attorneys who did much of this work. Outside recognition of the scope of the outbreak was delayed until May or

June 2017, when hundreds of incarcerated women had already suffered from scabies, and numerous court and sheriff's department staff were also seeking treatment.[7] But it appears the initial cases in this facility actually started a year earlier on the male side of the housing areas, in mid-2016, and the jump to the women's side occurred in late 2016.[8] Incarcerated people and their attorneys were able to identify a male prisoner who was among those with scabies in 2016 and who started a prison job as a trustee in late 2016, moving throughout the male and female housing areas. He reported submitting multiple sick-call requests that were ignored, including one expressly stating he thought he had scabies. He even submitted a WebMD printout on scabies. During this time "he complained about the rash that had spread over his body. He was falsely informed that he had 'contact dermatitis' or a reaction to 'something in the laundry.'"[9]

This work done by incarcerated people and their attorneys underscores an important aspect of many outbreaks behind bars: the denial of care to individuals goes hand in hand with ignoring the scope of the problem. It's often possible to look back and find very sophisticated letters and summaries of the early stages of an outbreak written by incarcerated people, and used as evidence by their attorneys, all because the facility staff and outside departments of health don't do this work as a routine part of health surveillance. In many cases, the facility and outsiders' pushback against admitting the problem is due to a fear of legal repercussions. In the cases of Ms. Snead and the other women who brought lawsuits, a federal judge ultimately decided that the problems faced by the women with scabies were experienced widely enough that all of the women could be certified as a class. This point in a legal case can receive lots of resistance, some of which is focused on the facility showing the problems aren't common or widespread, or there isn't any proof that incarcerated people followed the required procedures to seek care and report problems. Frequently, basic public-health principles of defining the full scope of an outbreak run headlong into the efforts of a facility or their lawyers to portray the problem as minimal, individual, or nonexistent.

***

Sometimes, an outside actor can really upset the normal dysfunction of outbreak responses in jails and prisons. Dr. Walter Barkey was such a disruptor in 2018. A dermatologist practicing in Flint, Michigan, Dr. Barkey heard through a friend that a loved one had been exposed to a scabies outbreak in Huron Valley, a women's prison. Dr. Barkey took the incredible step of cold calling the prison, offering his services, and then pushing to be let in to help respond to the outbreak. Although corrections officials would later try to present his efforts as something they sought, it is clear he heard about the outbreak and took the rare initiative as a community physician to push his way into the facility to see what was happening. In doing so, he brought technical and professional expertise to bear, but he also dramatically increased the profile of the outbreak to spotlight the lack of treatment for women in the facility. The *Detroit Free Press* chronicled his efforts, and he told their reporter that the public messaging of prison officials bringing him in wasn't correct: "Only after several phone interviews was my offer to come and see inmates at the facility accepted. . . . To my knowledge there were never any plans to 'bring in' a dermatologist."[10] Reporting on the outbreak also revealed the prison officials actually blamed incarcerated women themselves: "In early December, prison officials blamed inmates for the rash, theorizing it was caused by improper mixing of prison-issued cleaning fluids by inmate porters who are charged with cleaning the prison, along with an inmate practice of using homemade laundry detergent to hand-wash their brassieres and underwear, rather than sending them to the prison laundry."[11]

Like the scabies outbreak in Nashville with Ms. Snead, this one had been going on for almost a year without the for-profit company that provided health care initiating widespread treatment. Once Dr. Barkey came in and made his assessment of a scabies outbreak clear, the company relented and agreed to treat all 2,000 women in the facility. One lesson to take from Dr. Barkey's involvement is that when patients are being ignored behind bars, outside health staff can and should assist them, even when involvement isn't welcomed or sought. That same type of effort, often without support or payment, can be impactful across a range of public-health problems that often go ignored. Dr. Barkey had already used his skills to reveal another largely neglected public-health problem by conducting examinations for skin rashes in response to the Flint water crisis. In that work, Dr. Barkey and other dermatologists crafted a standardized survey tool and examination that they could use to evaluate skin rashes among Flint residents, whose water supply was potentially contaminated with both caustic chemicals and infectious agents.[12]

Another lesson from the Michigan scabies outbreak is that a lack of competent infection-control measures can have a drastic effect. Most jails and prisons have a role identified as infection-control officer, but I have often investigated outbreaks where this position simply hasn't been filled. This results in cost savings but leaves the facility without dedicated nursing staff to ensure proper measures are being followed.

For scabies, the intensity, history, and widespread nature of the rashes may not be enough to make a definitive diagnosis, although all these elements should raise a strong suspicion of a scabies outbreak. Diagnosis of individual patients is best accomplished by taking skin scrapings from affected areas of the patient's body and looking at those scrapings under a microscope.[13] Health departments and primary-care resources offer protocols for this step, but in an outbreak, it takes infection-control officers to ensure the right people are assessed in the correct manner. It seems as if the facility health staff were simply not led or directed to take these steps in Michigan. Dr. Barkey brought his microscope in to the prison so he could do this test on his own. The lack of training by facility staff to do the testing themselves was revealed by one of the prison's own nurses, who commented that "health officials at the prison, who had not received training in diagnosing scabies, were taking scrapings near where lesions were visible, but these were areas where the women had likely scratched and already removed the mites."[14]

In the lawsuit against CoreCivic in Nashville (the for-profit prison-management company), attorneys for the women reported the following:

> Despite a contractual obligation to employ staff to oversee infection control, CoreCivic has not employed anyone in those positions for at least one and possibly four years, and it does not use any procedure for screening inmates for scabies or other parasitic infections during intake. And, despite a contractual obligation to do so, it does not procure or review the medical records of inmates transferred to the facility who have special health care needs.[15]

This lack of resources for infection control affected efforts to diagnose and treat women with scabies, but it also brings us back to the man who was experiencing the same denials of treatment himself and then was approved to take a job as a trustee, moving around the facility without having gone through the basic infection-control assessments required for that position. The lawsuit mentioned this specific failure: "Although [redacted] did not receive a health screening or tuberculosis test upon entry, when he was appointed to a prison job as a 'trustee' a few months after his arrival, he was required to have a health screening."[16]

Examples of What Works

Both scabies outbreaks we've looked at offer insights into correctional facilities' efforts to hide problems from those who might pry from the outside. For example, the complaint in the Nashville case reported that

> in early July 2017, the defendant's Health Administrator
> falsely informed the inmates that no one at MDCDF had
> been diagnosed with scabies. Finally, on or around July 17,
> 2017, the Health Department visited the facility. Twelve
> inmates who had filed grievances about lack of medical
> treatment were placed in solitary before the Health Depart-
> ment's arrival and were unable to speak with Health
> Department representatives while they were there.[17]

Hiding or sequestering people away in solitary-confinement units is a common practice in jails and prisons, and it's painful to contemplate that health officials may have gone to investigate an outbreak and not sought out people in these places simply because they were led wherever the facility staff wanted them to go. Anyone who has been incarcerated or had a family member behind bars would likely know the standard set of precautions and preparations that occur when outside inspectors come into a facility. These can involve cleaning up, staffing up, moving people out of sight or earshot, painting the walls, and posting lots of new signs.

The scabies outbreaks also reveal another common tactic used to hide problems with health care from the outside world: the grievance process. Outside health officials often aren't aware that much of the relevant information about the onset and incidence of outbreak symptoms isn't in jail or prison medical records. Medical records will show when reports of symptoms are recognized and a patient is scheduled for care. But people who are ignored or denied care may have extensive documentation of when their symptoms arose and how they are feeling, all reported in medical grievances, which often go into an administrative silo. When people are detained, they are usually given an inmate handbook that lays out a dizzying set of rules about how medical problems should be reported through sick calls, and then if they aren't addressed, through filing a grievance. This approach exists partly because of the Prison Litigation Reform Act (PLRA), a federal law from 1996 that made it much harder for incarcerated people to file lawsuits about their treatment. A core element of the PLRA is the requirement that a person "exhaust their remedies," meaning they need to follow the rules about filing sick calls then grievances and then appeals, and if they don't follow each of these steps in order, then the facility can move to try to dismiss a lawsuit filed later because of their failure to follow the steps. These steps can take months or even years to resolve.[18]

Inside jails and prisons, each of these steps can be ignored by facility staff or replied to in a way that is slow or meaningless. As people get repeatedly dismissed trying to seek care, or receive nonsense replies to their grievances, they often just give up or miss a step in the process, creating an opportunity to have a lawsuit dismissed later on. This is a central feature of the PLRA, not a bug. Sick-call requests and grievances submitted by people during an outbreak are not even on the radar of most public-health staffers when they walk into a jail or prison, but they should be.[19] Following the scabies outbreak in Michigan, Rachell Garwood was one of the women who filed a lawsuit about the lack of care by the facility and Corizon Inc.[20] The facility tried to have the lawsuit dismissed in part because they said she hadn't exhausted her remedies for seeking care and trying to resolve the issues as required by the PLRA. Fortunately, the judge in this case saw the reality of what she had endured. Part of the opinion denying the request of the facility to dismiss her complaint included the following:

> Between January and March 2019, Garwood submitted at least six kite requests for medical treatment. Garwood filed a Step I grievance on March 7, 2019 after her sixth kite was unresolved and a rash on her arm continued to cause her pain. MDOC responded on April 22, 2019 by saying the Step I grievance was "resolved" since Garwood was seen by medical personnel on January 10, 2019. Garwood says health care officials cancelled her January 2019 appointment and never rescheduled. She did not receive the Step I response until May 15, 2019—more than two months after she submitted the grievance. Garwood appealed the Step I response on May 21, 2019. MDOC denied her Step II

grievance on June 5, 2019 for the same reason. Garwood's response—again—was she never received treatment because her appointment was canceled. Garwood appealed the Step II response; MDOC denied it on July 30, 2019. MDOC said that Garwood's "disagreement with the treatment plan does not constitute a denial of care." MDOC, again, contended the grievance was resolved because health care professionals saw Garwood on either January 10, 2019 or January 14, 2019. However, Garwood attests she never had a health care appointment.[21]

This decision by the judge, along with the original lawsuit, reveals just how much crucial information about an outbreak can be sequestered away from patient medical records. Fortunately, people who submit sick-call requests and grievances often have notes and original copies of their submissions. Facilities also have these records, but often the documents must be asked for separately from medical records.

***

A simple search of news articles for "scabies" and "jail" or "prison" yields dozens of recent examples.[22] The delays in care from facility staff as well as local health officials in these cases show a high level of comfort for prolonged suffering of incarcerated people. These delays are especially tolerated when the usually nonfatal ectoparasites lice and scabies are involved. Whatever the threshold is to motivate a speedy response, or to hold facilities responsible afterward, scabies outbreaks seem to fall well below that mark much of the time. Most of these cases, like the spectrum of other outbreaks behind bars, do not result in any lawsuits or trials that hold facilities to account for their failures. In addition, the consequences of these failures of basic infection control follow people home. The judge's ruling in the CoreCivic case in Nashville included reports from patients about the financial burden of retreatment when they arrived home and their inability to work in some cases because they were isolating at home.[23]

The simplest and most reliable way to avoid outbreaks behind bars is to not be incarcerated. This principle is especially true when the infectious agent is rarely detected or treated, like scabies. Aside from preventing exposure through incarceration, and promoting speedy response to cases when they arise, another important area of mitigation involves addressing poor sanitation. There are no enforced standards about how often living spaces, bathrooms, showers, and other parts of jails, prisons, and detention centers should be cleaned. This problem is complicated because, while health staff may detect an infection relating to poor sanitation or other conditions, it falls to the security service that controls the physical parts of the facility to do something about it. Even more complicated is the situation when cleaning is done by incarcerated people with few resources and little training, or when there's a dispute about who is supposed to clean something. In my first weeks at Rikers, a large seagull flew into the razor wire near the window of my trailer office, and the dead body of the ensnared bird started to smell badly within a day or two. When I called around to see if there was someone who could remove it, I entered a rotation of calls and referrals that left me without any answers. So the quickest resolution was to let the body completely fall apart and decompose. I stepped into a long-term version of this sanitation quandary when an EMT showed me an air vent covered with an inch of mold. The vent was in a room where newly arrested people were screened for health problems before they went into Manhattan court pens to wait for arraignment and either release or transfer to jail. The EMTs who did this important job, finding people who might die without care in the coming hours, worked in two cramped rooms the size of walk-in closets. The EMTs said the vent had never been cleaned and pointed out that they and the patients they screened sat under this air vent that looked more like a section of black shag carpet or a velvet Elvis poster than anything circulated air could pass through. The EMTs had reported this vent to their supervisors for years but to no avail. As I tracked the path of people from arrest and transport by the police department to this room, staffed by New York City fire department EMTs, then to the pens staffed by the city's department of corrections and up to the courts run by New York's Office of Court Administration, in a building owned by one city agency and maintained and inspected by another, the yearslong struggle to get this vent cleaned became numbingly clear.

The plight of the EMTs and the people being screened in this room showed me how a serious sanitation problem could be impossible to address when minimum standards of care aren't applied. I can think of many patient-care spaces in jails and prisons I've been in since that were filthy, infested with vermin, too hot, too cold, or otherwise not adequate for providing basic medical care.[24]

These kinds of problems with sanitation also include access to laundry services and showers behind bars. Both laundry and showers are prescribed by institutional polices, but in reality, how often they are actually available varies greatly. In some minimum- and medium-security environments, people have access to laundry machines and dryers on their housing units, but the norm is a central laundry operation that collects linens and clothes from all housing areas and sends them back once or twice per week. Many people have only a single towel, which they often wash and try to dry in their cell or dorm bunk. When laundry services are interrupted, more pieces of clothes and linens must be washed in the housing area or cell sinks, leading to less thorough clearing of scabies and other infectious agents.

The two scabies outbreaks discussed in this chapter show how simply listening to people who present with new health problems and then initiating basic medical and public-health responses can make a meaningful difference—and reduce illness and pain.

Recommendations

- Seek written communications (sick-call slips, grievances, letters) and internal facility emails regarding the outbreak for health-department review as early as possible.
- Ensure outside health-department staff and specialists have face-to-face, confidential encounters with people who are reporting these problems.
- Review the infection-control staffing and resources available to manage the outbreak inside the facility. This includes learning who the full-time equivalents of infection-control nurses are that have worked during the current and recent pay periods.[25]
- Assess costs for people returning home following an outbreak, including the cost of medications (about $50 for the first tube of permethrin for scabies treatment) and delays to starting work because they need to isolate, and the cost of laundry services.

- If there is an inspection of the facility, take efforts to gather meaningful information, not simply the version of events the facility wants to present.

Research ideas

- Hypothesis: Access to treatment for scabies and lice outbreaks behind bars is often inadequate. Approach: Review facility data on detection and treatment of an outbreak; compare with grievance and sick-call requests for outbreak symptoms. Review lawsuits that may provide information in this area.[26]
- Hypothesis: Facility staff often fail to provide treatment in hand or prescriptions for people returning home during a scabies or lice outbreak. Approach: Interview currently or formerly incarcerated people after scabies and lice outbreaks to learn about their access to care and the financial costs they experienced after going home.

CHAPTER SEVEN

Independent Inspections During Outbreaks

etting into the Memphis jail felt like descending into the New York City subway. Underground escalators led to a long, dark central hallway with even darker cell blocks off to either side. Down at the end of the main hallway were a couple of units, directly across from each other. One of these was apparently where people with active COVID-19 were being held. This inspection was in the summer of 2020, so the basic risks of COVID-19 were known, but there was no vaccine yet.[1] I'd driven to Memphis from New York because flying didn't seem safe. I had already done six facility COVID-19 inspections, including Cook County Jail in Chicago. Along the way, I'd developed a plan for how to conduct an inspection, including what PPE (personal protective equipment) I would need and what other precautions to take to minimize risk to myself as well as the people I was around.

There in the Memphis jail, in Shelby County, I made my way from the intake area to the medical clinic and various housing areas, leaving the ones used for people with active

COVID-19 last. As I worked down the long hallway toward the COVID-19 unit, I went into the cell blocks for newly admitted people, which were along small offshoots of the main hallway. Down each of these cramped offshoots was a narrow passageway and a few barred cells beyond. Just opening the door and walking into the low-ceilinged hallway brought a rush of yells, as well as a powerful blast of the aromas of urine, feces, and vomit. Three years after my visit, a man with serious mental illness named Gershun Freeman was held in one of these cells, and when the door was opened, he rushed out, was restrained and beaten by 10 officers, had an officer kneel on his back for almost six minutes, and died. The video of his death gives a sense of how filthy and violent these small spaces can be, as well as the underlying tragedy of untreated mental illness in jails.[2] During my inspection, these tiny areas struck me more like police holding cells than real housing areas. The low ceilings and cramped quarters made it clear that COVID-19 would quickly pass from one person to another, especially since the jail had not instituted routine testing upon admission.

Moving down the larger hallway, I kept looking for medical isolation signs, a PPE cart, or other telltale indications to point me to the unit where people with active COVID-19 were housed. At the end of the hallway, there were just two units left, both of which had doors with bars in them. On one side, the unit was quiet, and on the other, a person could be heard screaming unintelligibly. I asked a corrections officer where I could find the medical isolation unit and was told it was right where we were standing—it was the quiet unit behind the door with the bars. None of the officers seemed to have the right level of PPE for this area. As I stepped aside to swap my KN95 mask for my own fit-tested N95 mask and other

PPE, I gave my customary disclaimer to the group around me, saying I was happy to proceed alone onto the unit and would be speaking with people and taking notes for a while. Some of the group stayed back, but some came with me, and I didn't see any of them taking extra precautions to enter the isolation area.

Inside the housing section, the individual cells had solid doors, but many of them had broken plexiglass windows, and some people were out of their cells in the open area between them. It was clear that little would impede the virus from passing to staff in the hallway outside this unit and to the housing area across the hall, especially with all the yelling. This realization was alarming enough that I made specific mention of the potential for transmission in my report:

> I am extremely concerned that anyone in the hallway outside 2A is routinely exposed to COVID-19 and would recommend testing of all staff and detainees who have been in this vicinity. This would include patients and staff who have been in the mental health unit 2N. These deficiencies are even more concerning given mounting evidence that the COVID-19 virus persists and travels in the air for longer than originally thought.[3]

When I inspected the quarantine units where people with potential exposure to COVID-19 were being kept apart from nonquarantined people, I saw a similar problem: "At the time of my inspection, two of three adjacent housing areas, 5b and 5c, were on quarantine because of previously identified cases. Unit 5a was not on quarantine. The front of all three units come together in a small, shared hallway, with open bars that allow for free movement of air (and virus) into and out of the three units."[4]

My report on the outbreak response in this facility found both strengths and areas for improvement, but few of them would have been evident without a physical inspection. For example, when I inspected the intake area, the people going through their booking and initial jail admission steps were all sitting with empty seats between them. While this spacing could have been done just for my inspection, this kind of social-distancing effort was not made in numerous other COVID-19 jail inspections I did.

Case Study Analysis

My independent inspection of the Memphis jail occurred because of a lawsuit filed about COVID-19 responses. I was retained by the ACLU as part of their work to seek protection for medically vulnerable people in the Shelby County Jail who were at heightened risk of death from COVID-19.[5] My own experience during this inspection showed me that many steps had already been taken by the facility staff to address basic issues around treatment and preventing morbidity and mortality; but like most jails and prisons, there hadn't been an independent medical review of how well or complete these efforts were. The closed nature of carceral settings almost predetermines a potentially severe disconnect between the reality experienced by detained people and the official account of what is happening. This difference, plus preexisting problems in the health services, can create a strong disincentive to do any objective assessment of an outbreak status and response.

In the Shelby County case, learning the reality of how or whether high-risk people were being protected required seeing the physical spaces and speaking with staff and detained people. Aside from the issues with transmission risk I mentioned above, my interviews with people who had COVID-19 revealed that on the isolation unit, nurses would check on each person daily—on weekdays. No checks were conducted from Friday afternoon until Monday morning. This was a terrifying thing to learn given how quickly people with COVID-19 (especially those with preexisting risk factors) can deteriorate. This type of gap in care can be fixed but needs to be identified and then given resources, such as allocating weekend nursing staff to do regular checks. These deficiencies in the Shelby County Jail, either not seen or not addressed by staff, are examples of why we need independent inspections of these settings, and why we need to anchor those inspections in visual observations, and conversations with detained people and staff, and not simply rely on the reports of facility leaders.

A correctional expert named Mike Brady also conducted inspections of this facility at the request of the court. His reports, like mine, relied heavily on his ability to see the physical areas of the jail and to speak with people who worked there and were detained there.[6] About six months after my inspection, and following many legal motions by both sides, the county entered into an agreement with the plaintiffs stating it would take several important steps to protect high-risk people during the COVID-19 pandemic, including some expedited releases of high-risk people, more outside monitoring, and improved ventilation and other mitigation efforts.[7]

Although in the Shelby County case, the ACLU was able to convince the judge of the need for outside inspection of the facility, my experience is that in most circumstances this idea is quickly objected to by whoever runs the facility. And the way the objection plays out is unpredictable. I encountered this issue, about a month before my Shelby inspection, when working with the Southern Poverty Law Center to document the inadequacies of the COVID-19 response in two notorious immigration detention centers, Stewart and Irwin, both in Georgia. Attorneys for the Department of Homeland Security argued the inspections were unwarranted and too disruptive, given the focus on COVID-19. In this instance, the federal judge agreed and mandated that the only possible inspections would be remote. I'd already made the case that this would not be sufficient and would amount to more of a guided video tour than an inspection, but with no alternative available, I proceeded.

The video inspections were problematic in several respects. First, I was unable to have brief conversations with detained people as I worked through the inspections—conversations which were crucial to understanding whether facility policies like symptom screening for COVID-19 or access to chronic-care appointments were actually occurring. Second, the nature of following someone carrying an iPad or other camera means the viewer can see only what's directly in front of the camera, in the 5–10 feet of the foreground. The inspector can't see anything the camera isn't pointing to. In one instance I reported, I saw an obvious issue farther away that I needed to inspect, but when I asked to see in that direction, the camera was quickly pointed to a wall to show off new signage. When the camera panned back to where I had requested, the issue had vanished. This was my first experience doing a video inspection, and I found that in circumstances when the facts of the outbreak response are in dispute, which is clearly the case in litigation, it is inadequate.

During an outbreak, the exact role of an outside inspector largely depends on the way the inspection came to pass. For example, when a group of detained people brings a lawsuit about their treatment during an outbreak, their attorneys may hire a medical expert to conduct an inspection of the facility. The facility will almost always object to this inspection, and a judge will decide whether it can occur. The two sets of attorneys will negotiate the terms of the inspection, and this is where the objections to speaking with detained people or staff, or having access to some parts of the facility or its data will come into play. It may be that both the facility and the detained people hire their own experts in response to a plaintiff's expert. I've done plenty of inspections alongside medical experts hired by ICE or the US Bureau of Prisons, and not surprisingly, they do not find the same problems I do.

For example, in the case above where I was blocked from doing an in-person inspection at two facilities, the Department of Homeland Security hired a physician to be their expert in this matter who opined that a video inspection was fine. He reported, "Contrary to Dr. Venters' experience detailed in his report, where he noted that the 'virtual inspection is a completely inadequate substitute for an in-person inspection,' I found it to be more than satisfactory."[8] He found the video inspection to be not only sufficient but to reveal well-functioning health-care systems inside Stewart and Irwin detention centers. He opined, "It is my opinion that both facilities have achieved large-scale implementation success. They have also clearly demonstrated organizational commitment to modifying such best practices as further information is learned and additional guidance is developed."[9] It is worth noting that shortly after our video inspections, a whistleblower came forward, a nurse who worked in one of the facilities, reporting serious failures in COVID-19 responses—exactly the kinds of issues that would be sought through in-person inspection and conversations with staff and detained people.[10] ICE would ultimately close down the Stewart detention center based on problems with health care, sexual abuse, and retaliation against women who had reported problems.[11] But in the middle of the COVID-19 outbreak, ICE and the for-profit facility were able to prevail with the judge in forcing a video inspection as opposed to a more rigorous in-person one.

Sometimes a judge may decide to avoid this dueling-expert problem and retain someone to inspect a facility and report back to the court on the outbreak response. I had this role in three inspections at the federal prison in Lompoc, California. Because this role stems from a judge wanting to get the unvarnished truth and clear recommendations, the inspector can request pretty much any data or access relevant to the role. For me, this included conducting numerous interviews with incarcerated people and staff as well as reviewing medical records of people who'd died from COVID-19. A significant part of my findings and recommendations focused on the inadequacies in how the Bureau of Prisons reviews deaths.

The work in these inspections usually involves a split between walking through the facility and speaking with people along the way. The rules of the inspection agreement can provide plenty of friction. For example, facility attorneys may direct their staff not to answer questions if they think the inspector is asking something outside the approved scope. Conversations with health staff can be even trickier when they work for a for-profit vendor and the vendor's attorneys don't want the inspector to speak with the staff. This can lead to long and combative days if there is a basic disconnect about what the inspection agreement includes. On one of my early inspections, a dispute over who could ask questions of the detained people quickly escalated to a dispute between at-torneys and a call to the judge for resolution.

Most of the time in my inspections, I simply note whether a question that seems important to the outbreak response is not answered. A good example is the use of sick call. Facility attorneys may say that asking staff about the sick-call process isn't related to COVID-19 because it's just part of the regular health system. But if making a sick call is the way people report their COVID-19 symptoms, then this objection doesn't make sense. I faced similar objections to asking about access to chronic care, but again, poorly treated chronic health problems increase the risk of death from COVID-19 and other infectious diseases; so, while it's directly relevant to the adequacy of the outbreak response, there is often no end to the ways the attorneys for the facilities can object to an outsider seeking information. Conversely, when the facility and their attorneys are on the same page about wanting to show off their efforts and make more improvements, these types of objections don't happen, and the attorneys may be hearing directly from staff about strengths and challenges for the first time.

The logistics of these inspections usually involve a short meeting with leadership in the morning, then agreeing on a route of physical spaces to see and how conversations can happen with staff and detained people. In larger prisons and jails, which may have multiple facilities and up to 7,500 people in custody, it can require several days to understand the risks of the outbreak and how the facility response is working. Many of the areas for improvement in these larger systems involve the ways in which people move into and around the facilities. For example, as people go to and from court in county jails, they are usually taken from their housing areas and put into pens at the intake of the jail. There, they may be crammed in close contact with people for up to an hour. While facilities will have some policy about social distancing in these settings, it's important to see what these pens look like while being used, and to understand whether or how the facility does contact tracing that includes time in one of these pens. A paradoxical gap often exists for people who need infirmary level of care because of illness or who need to be admitted to the mental-health unit of the jail or prison. In these circumstances, the basic precautions for outbreak prevention and response may not be followed. For example, I've inspected many facilities with a sound practice of intake quarantine and testing for most newly arrived people, but they would simply skip these steps for people with serious mental illness or those who were going through detoxification, placing them onto specialized units for these health issues alongside others who hadn't recently arrived. This practice has been more prevalent for women, often because of a lack of space and staffing allotted to their care.

Examples of What Works

One of the most predictable aspects of an inspection is the way a facility prepares to put on a good face. Most often, this involves extensively cleaning the facility in the days before the inspector arrives, and sometimes painting walls and doors as well. There may also be a quick effort to get basic sanitation and hygiene issues addressed, with more soap, paper towels, and access to laundry, and even increased medical care. Another common preparation is to print and laminate massive amounts of new signage. These measures are fairly common, and even when not so obvious, detained people are quick to report them. All of this highlights the need for unannounced inspections, which are standard in nursing homes, hospitals, and ambulatory care settings but not in most prisons and jails.

A primary concern for the inspector is the real risk of retaliation against people who offer their insights and experiences. In about a third of the inspections I've done, the people I spoke with were concerned about retaliation in the form of verbal or physical abuse. Detained people know these risks far better than I do, and while an inspector can address these threats or acts in a report, the reality is that by stepping forward to report the truth, detained people (and sometimes staff) risk many types of retaliation. This might take the form of having a person's cell "tossed"; meaning, security staff rip pictures and other things off the wall and throw out anything they deem contraband, including clothing, bedding, or medications. Or retaliation may include being beaten or placed into a small cage for hours while restrained.

The problem of retaliation can be improved with more regular inspections and especially with unannounced inspections on nights and weekends, when correctional and health supervisors are often scarce and retaliation can occur more easily. But during an outbreak, the facility leadership may be acutely worried about presenting an "everything is fine here" image to the public and may seek to silence voices of dissent among detained people or staff. On the other hand, I have been in many facilities where the leadership were genuinely seeking help with their response. This attitude often reflects a leadership style that seeks to find problems and address them both to resolve the outbreak and to be transparent. Of course, leaders like wardens and superintendents are not the ones in housing areas at night or on the weekend. One of the chronic issues that allows abuse and neglect to persist behind bars is that correctional leaders who seek to improve conditions may not work in a facility for more than a year or two, making it difficult for them to identify and address staff who engage in abusive practices or to understand the systems that promote them, like solitary confinement.

Jails, prisons, and immigration detention systems routinely fight to keep independent inspectors out of their facilities, and the COVID-19 pandemic provided a popular rationale for these objections. Facilities sowing fear about how outside inspectors would import and spread COVID-19 is something I encountered frequently, although the concern was usually dismissed once judges reviewed the evidence available to them, notwithstanding the ICE case involving the Stewart and Irwin detention centers. I was asked to help with such an objection in Alabama, where the state's Department of Corrections (ADOC) was arguing that a psychiatrist who had been performing inspections to determine compliance with mental-health standards for prisons shouldn't be allowed into the facilities. The Alabama prison system has a well-documented history of problems with mental-health services, which the judge in the case characterized as "horrendously inadequate."[12] The judge further stated, "Despite its knowledge of actual harm and substantial risks of serious harm to mentally ill prisoners, ADOC has failed to respond reasonably to identified issues in the delivery of mental health care."[13] So having an independent expert conduct these checks on mental health care was truly a critical function for incarcerated people. But the prison system tried to block the inspections during COVID-19 with the incredible assertion that "no court has ever sanctioned this form of 'super spreader' site touring through multiple facilities."[14]

I had been doing COVID-19 inspections for many months and was even finishing up two days of inspections in the nearby Mississippi prison system when I got the call to help with this case. A hearing was called in which the mental-health expert explained the extensive infection-control precautions she would take to follow CDC guidelines, and I testified about my work conducting inspections safely during the COVID-19 pandemic. The ADOC retained a physician to give the opinion that these inspections shouldn't occur, but even he ultimately agreed during the hearing that outside inspections are important. The judge in the case dismissed the ADOC efforts to block the psychiatrist's access and ruled the inspections could proceed. Importantly, the judge made clear that the efforts of the prison system to substitute confidential, in-person interviews with remote telemedicine were not appropriate, ruling, "The court further finds that the telemedicine interviews of prisoners proposed by defendants' expert are not an adequate substitute for the confidential interviews of prisoners proposed by [the physician], as the defendants presented no evidence that the prisoners could be assured of confidentiality with the telemedicine option."[15] This was a small win, but it was significant given the substantial energy the ADOC had put into blocking transparency about a problem that had already been established.

***

Some of the most thorough inspections I've been a part of were those conducted by the Civil Rights Division of the US Department of Justice (DOJ). I was happy to start working with them several years ago on a case in the Massachusetts state prison system that focused on how people with serious mental illness were being placed into conditions that were essentially solitary confinement but were labeled as "mental health watch."[16] These kinds of investigations often occur when the Civil Rights Division of the DOJ and a local US attorney team up to investigate especially serious allegations about how a jail or prison is operating. My first exposure to the depth of their work occurred when the DOJ launched an investigation into brutality at Rikers Island. I was the medical director there at the time and our team was eager to supply them with data on injuries among our patients due to use of force, data we had been sharing with security leadership without much impact.[17] Because these are legal investigations, they may span a year or more just to collect data, conduct facility inspections, do interviews, and write reports. This depth and pace mean that a DOJ investigation may not translate into a quick improvement for people inside the system. And the ultimate outcome of most of these investigations—usually a settlement agreeing on how the facility or system will improve conditions and stop violating the rights of detained people—may prove very difficult to achieve. In the New York City jails, for example, the original case led to a settlement with the DOJ and the monitor assigned to ensure the city's Department of Correction addresses violence and brutality. The monitor issued about 25 reports over eight years that showed things had not improved and that his confidence in the city's willingness to make these changes was evaporating, which led the judge in the case to hold New York City in contempt.[18] This lack of change in New York may eventually lead to something called "receivership," where the federal judge takes control of the jails away from the city and gives it to a receiver who runs the system—an extreme outcome that shows the city has failed repeatedly and isn't likely to improve.[19] Conversely, when both sides agree on a path toward improvements, the thoroughness of the DOJ investigations can yield specific and trackable steps to make lasting improvements to care.

So, while thorough, these DOJ investigations are slow moving and not a great model for outbreak responses. At the core of this approach is the legal context of the DOJ's inspections, which is to build the case that a system exhibits a "pattern or practice" of violating the constitutional rights of people in its custody.[20] This notion really gets at the heart of our national failure regarding correctional health. While each DOJ investigation is thorough and is a reliable approach to documenting serious lapses in care or other elements of incarceration that rise to the level of a denial of civil rights, the process is slower moving and more limited in scope than structures that monitor health care in community settings. We have lots of mandated inspections of hospitals, nursing homes, and other settings by state and federal health agencies as well as accrediting bodies like the Joint Commission. These organizations look at infection control as well as the full breadth of health services provided. Depending on the organization, systemic failures are met with suspended or terminated licenses to operate, or threats to funding and reimbursement for repeatedly inadequate assessments. For example, the federal agency Centers for Medicare and Medicaid Services (CMS) can threaten to withhold all its funding that goes to a hospital. A recent report on hospitals with CMS's "immediate jeopardy" status found that, in 2022, 19 hospitals held this type of status and that, over 10 years, about 700 hospitals had received the designation. This report lays out how serious deficiencies, including preventable deaths, can trigger unannounced inspections and force corrective action plans to be implemented before the threat to a health facility's Medicaid and Medicare funding is reversed.[21]

Behind bars, there are a couple of pseudo-accrediting organizations in correctional health: the National Commission of Correctional Health Care (NCCHC) and the American Correctional Association (ACA). These groups have standards regarding the broad areas of health provision, but they lack the teeth of the community structures noted above. They are not true accrediting bodies in that participation is voluntary.[22] As a result, their standards are not enforced in a manner that means noncompliance leads to loss of service capacity or funding—unless a county or state makes having this accreditation mandatory with their for-profit vendors. These groups do conduct facility inspections and give internal audits to the facility about its deficiencies needing corrective actions. But one of the dismal parts of jail- and prison-death investigations is coming across years-old reports that were simply ignored.

The speed and lethality of outbreaks behind bars reveal the dire need for independent inspections. COVID-19 and other outbreaks have also made clear that, in many facilities, the presence of an outbreak can be quickly leveraged to reduce transparency under the guise of infection-control concerns. We rely on lawsuits and the decisions of judges to generate inspections because our nation lacks a framework for mandated independent inspections of jails, prisons, and immigration detention centers. This lack is true for health care as well as general conditions of confinement, which impact health greatly and are also where deficiencies are commonly found. The need for mandated inspections is well-established around the world, and a standardized approach to this work exists in the Optional Protocol to the Convention Against Torture (OPCAT). This treaty, which was established in 2002 and came into effect in 2006, builds on the principles established in the actual Convention Against Torture by fleshing out how each nation will prevent torture behind bars by setting up structures that independently monitor detention settings.[23] The United States is a party to the original convention, but never signed or ratified the Optional Protocol, and is thus not among the 90 nations that have committed to this approach.[24] In nations that have adopted this approach, both governmental and nonprofit organizations conduct and support independent inspections. One of these groups, Dignity—Danish Institute Against Torture, has not only conducted this type of work at home but has helped other nations develop their own monitoring systems. Dignity also created an extremely useful manual for health professionals about monitoring places of detention that not only outlines the various purposes of this type of monitoring but also provides granular details on how it can be conducted.[25] This approach can be found across the nations where the Optional Protocol has been adopted, but it is nonexistent here in the United States.

Instead of a national commitment to independent inspection and monitoring of detention settings in the United States, we have a patchwork of local and state efforts to replicate some of these principles, with a predictably muted impact. Some states have created commissions or boards that oversee or inspect prisons or jails, as is the case in New York with the Commission on Correction and the local Board of Correction in New York City. In California, the state attorney general has created a mechanism to inspect immigration detention settings and report on conditions and adequacy of care, while separate efforts are focused on jails and prisons, often including investigations of civil-rights violations by state attorneys general and the US Department of Justice.

One area of promise from my standpoint is the emergence of disability-rights groups. These nonprofit organizations have state mandates to protect the rights of disabled people, and in many states, they've taken on an increasing role in calling out abuse and neglect behind bars.[26] Some of the COVID-19 inspections I've done have been with state disability-rights organizations, and I've seen how they have good access to people and data because of their existing legal mandate as a "protection and advocacy" group.[27] In Arizona and Florida, I worked with state disability-rights groups to inspect both jails and state psychiatric hospitals during outbreaks. Because of the ongoing presence of those advocacy workers in these facilities, and their mandate to have access, the inspections were more collegial, and facility staff focused more on providing technical assistance than I experienced during some of the litigation inspections.

One goal of justice reform should absolutely include adoption of OPCAT so we can create a national structure of detention monitoring linked to standards and practices from around the world. This requires congressional action as well as leadership from the president. But this effort need not slow local and regional progress to build on the small number of inspections we currently have. There are a few other steps that can help promote independent inspections during outbreaks.

First, the disability-rights organizations in each state should be a point of contact and collaboration for the state department of health. These groups can share information about the status of outbreaks and health services. In some states, monitoring bodies like the John Howard Association of Illinois and the Correctional Association of New York are also important contacts for state health departments. In addition, some states and counties have dedicated oversight boards. The more that state health departments can meet with these groups conducting inspections before or at the outset of outbreaks, the less the departments will be reliant on facility administrators for their only perspective.

Whenever a state or county epidemiologist or other outside expert does conduct an inspection during an outbreak, there should be a readout of their assessment with some of these groups to validate their conclusions. This is especially true when the facility requests input on management of an outbreak and then arranges for the entire visit with little or no contact with detained people. The more the voices of people living through the outbreak are incorporated into the assessment done by outside inspectors, the more accurate their findings will be and the more relevant their recommendations. A more concrete guide on how outsiders can approach inspections can be found in the last chapter of this book.

A second step to improving the quality and frequency of independent inspections would be to create state working groups that combine all the organizations conducting facility inspections. This type of working group already exists for coordinating services after release from prison and jail in many cities, but a coalition that also includes state and local health departments would provide a structure to standardize how the adequacy of care is assessed. This structure would be especially helpful during outbreaks and would bring together the perspectives of facility administrators, detained people and their families, and local public-health staff. This type of working group can also include advocacy and academic partners to help with data analysis that would review mortality during outbreaks and then publish that data. Two groups in California, the UCLA COVID Behind Bars Data Project and the Amend group at UCSF, have done some of this vital work, but we need to grow these efforts in every state, with a focus on independent inspections of local, state, and federal carceral settings. As well, a working group that pulls together the entities with a current legal mandate and other cohorts that can help with specific elements of an outbreak would be a great step forward.

When an outbreak does occur behind bars, these groups can work together with the prisons and jails to propose a more standardized approach to inspections. In Connecticut, a COVID-19 lawsuit led to a settlement between the State Department of Correction, which includes jails and prisons, and lawyers from the ACLU representing detained people. The settlement created a monitoring body—named the McPherson Panel for Tre McPherson, a man who'd been in jail because he couldn't pay his bond and subsequently developed COVID-19.[28] I was one of five people named to this body; each side in the lawsuit named two experts, and the four of us then picked a fifth. We spent approximately six months inspecting the Connecticut facilities, reviewing data, and writing reports on the adequacy of the state's efforts to implement CDC guidelines.[29] While there were some limitations to this approach, including a lack of access to some of the crucial mortality data I requested, it is a model that can be developed quickly. I served on a similar monitoring group in Hawaii's prisons and jails.[30] In future outbreaks, this approach can be implemented either as part of settlements or when governors and mayors want to promote transparency and evidence-based responses before they are forced into doing so by litigation.

Because the United States is one of the few wealthy nations without a framework for independent inspection of jails, prisons, and immigration detention centers, every crisis serves the dual purpose of reminding us of why we need inspections during outbreaks and offering a new opportunity for carceral systems to strip away what little transparency exists. As I've noted, most correctional settings have little or no routine inspection of the adequacy of health services provided to detained people, and when an outbreak starts, under the guise of infection control, there is a reflexive effort to shut down whatever inspections were occurring. When correctional settings do enlist outside experts, it often involves a narrow selection of infectious-disease experts without correctional experience, who deliver a finely tailored message about potential improvements, which can gloss over any systemic problems in health care or custodial practices inside the facilities. A first step toward increasing the frequency and value of facility inspections involves lawmakers and health departments validating and informing their work by seeking the counsel of groups that already advocate for incarcerated people.

Recommendations

- Oversight boards and organizations seeking transparency in carceral settings should always include inspections from outside experts as part of their assessment of the adequacy of a facility or system. These can be long-term authorities like the New York City BOC, or they can be time- and content-limited to outbreak response efforts.

- Inspections for non-outbreak reasons should not be halted during an outbreak, especially when the outside inspectors are medical professionals who can follow infection-control plans.
- Outside inspections should always include confidential interviews with detained people and staff. See the inspection guide in the appendix.

Research ideas

- Hypothesis: In-person inspections capture more thorough information about outbreaks behind bars than video inspections. Approach: Compare expert reports from plaintiffs, defendants, and independent experts on their assessments of outbreak responses. Compare these observations to those of the Joint Commission and state department of health inspection reports. Review lawsuits that may provide information in this area.[31]

CHAPTER EIGHT

Saving Lives During Outbreaks

The release of 74-year-old Gwen Levi from federal prison is a great example of what works in responding to outbreaks behind bars. Her case during the COVID-19 pandemic also shows just how easily a sound public-health policy can be ruined by the many trip wires of the criminal justice system. Early in the outbreak, the US Department of Justice took the important step of reviewing high-risk people for possible home confinement. Ms. Gwen Levi, a cancer survivor and grandmother, was released to home confinement after serving 16 years for a drug charge. She moved to Baltimore to live with her family, and one day, she didn't answer a call from her parole officer because she was taking a computer class. This lack of response led the Bureau of Prisons to consider her an escapee, and she was detained again. A judge quickly ordered her release, but her case drew swift national attention to the possibility that people who were thriving at home with their families could be returned to prison.[1] Ms. Levi and I both testified to the US House Judiciary Committee on this topic, and what struck me about her testimony was the incredible anxiety the experience had caused her, not knowing whether she would get COVID-19 and die in prison or how she could qualify for home confinement, and then being put through numerous confusing and contradictory orders regarding her freedom.

Case Study Analysis

The stories of Ms. Levi and others on home confinement from the BOP would not have made it to mainstream awareness without the advocacy of the nonprofits FAMM (Families Against Mandatory Minimums) and JustLeadershipUSA, organizations that advocate for reform led by people directly impacted by the criminal justice system. Their efforts were joined by US Senators Dick Durbin and Cory Booker, and the plight of these 4,500 individuals who were released but in jeopardy of being sent back to prison became a national discussion, tagged #Keepthemathome. Ultimately, the Department of Justice came to the decision that people could remain at home, not only resolving their personal uncertainty but also helping to keep federal prisons a bit less crowded for the sake of outbreak management.

Examples of What Works

The release of people from detention is the most powerful public-health intervention to prevent illness and death from large-scale outbreaks behind bars. There are plenty of more narrow and technical steps that are crucial for lowering risk during an outbreak, but we've learned over and over that release has the capacity to save lives. The benefits of release are twofold. First, by identifying and releasing high-risk people ahead of time, facilities can dramatically reduce the risk of death even when sustained transmission of infection occurs.

Second, for most outbreaks, including COVID-19, there is a need to separate sick people from exposed people, and to create spaces for newly arrived and soon-to-leave people. All of this reduces transmission but also groups people in cohorts based on the type of health precautions and tasks needed. These are fairly basic parts of outbreak management, but when facilities are above 75% of their capacity, even basic requirements become impossible to meet. The problem of a lack of space is especially apparent when people become ill and need infirmary level of care inside the facilities, or they need a hospital transfer. Most jails and prisons have small infirmaries that are usually filled with sick patients and cannot be emptied to care for multiple patients ill with COVID-19 or another highly contagious disease. For patients who are infected but asymptomatic, moving to a regular housing area being used for medical isolation may suffice, but the sicker the patients, the less space and fewer staff there are to care for them. And this problem becomes even more acute when patients need to be transferred to the hospital, where they will be accompanied by two armed correctional staff 24/7 and where space is also extremely tight. Consequently, the benefits of release during an outbreak are targeted toward patients who are most likely to die or require hospitalization, freeing up community resources as well.

There's another benefit of having fewer people in a jail or prison: blunting the power of the facility to serve as an engine of transmission that extends to the surrounding community. With highly transmissible infections like MRSA, TB, and COVID-19, incarceration drives transmission behind bars, which then spreads to many other people in surrounding communities. Dr. Eric Reinhart, an anthropologist and physician, conducted crucial research into the ways incarceration

drives community spread of COVID-19. He and his colleagues looked at the churn of people in and out of Chicago's
jail system and found that in March 2020 as the pandemic
exploded, almost 16% of cases in the entire state were driven
by Chicago jail incarcerations.[2] This dynamic involves the
jail acting as a kind of infection accelerator that exposes
both staff and incarcerated people, with the staff going home
to their families and communities every day and the incarcerated people going to court, home, and sometimes to prison.
Dr. Reinhart's team found each jail case could be linked to
five community cases, truly showing the multiplier effect that
incarceration has on infection.[3] They also found these jail-
driven cases served to dramatically widen the overall racial
disparities in the COVID-19 pandemic. The sheriff's department responded to these analyses by insulting the researchers, stating that "Mr. Reinhart's baseless and irresponsible
conclusion stands in stark contrast to the independent findings of the CDC, Yale, and Stanford Universities who concluded the practices implemented at the Cook County Jail to
contain the global pandemic collectively served as a model for
other carceral facilities to follow and prevented thousands of
cases and saved dozens of lives."[4] This response is classic for
correctional settings, where there is scant will to acknowledge
the health risks of incarceration. It's entirely possible that the
Cook County Jail was lauded by some for their COVID-19
efforts and simultaneously that the jail was a powerful accelerator of infection inside the facilities and in the surrounding community. One of the early facility inspections I
conducted was of this jail, having driven out from New York
before it felt safe to fly. I found both strengths and deficiencies in their response, but none of those specific observations
weaken the analyses of Dr. Reinhart and his colleagues.

By comparison, the possibility that outbreaks inside a facility can drive cases on the outside is well established when we think about infections driven by hospitalization. For example, the bacterial infection *Clostridium difficile* can cause deadly diarrhea and often occurs shortly after medical treatment and hospitalization. Research into how this infection is driven by hospitalization doesn't cause hospital administrators to label public-health researchers' work "baseless and irresponsible" but instead causes health agencies (including those in Cook County and the rest of Illinois) to partner with hospitals to reduce infections and track incidence data.[5] When the reality that infections behind bars drive community cases is denied, release of incarcerated people is off the table as a potential mitigation tool, and focus is forced onto only the steps taken inside the facility.

Overcrowding behind bars is a core risk factor for many types of bad health outcomes, including physical and behavioral health. Despite numerous successful lawsuits and settlements over the past 30 years regarding overcrowding, people in American carceral facilities are often held in numbers that exceed 100% or even 175% of the stated capacity.[6] The sleeping spaces in cells and dorms alike force close contact with others, as do the showers, sinks, toilets, and common areas for eating, programs, and recreation. I won't spend too much time on why overcrowding is bad for outbreak prevention and control other than to state the obvious: the close proximity is a core contributor to easy spread of viral, bacterial, and fungal infections, and the filth and lack of sanitation and hygiene also drive infections, especially the ectoparasites lice and scabies.

Overcrowding behind bars prevents a common tool for controlling outbreaks: social distancing. When the CDC put out their guidelines on COVID-19 in March 2020, they stated social distancing was important to prevent the spread of the virus behind bars,[7] but the design and operations of these facilities seem to make this impossible at times. Looking at three activities can help us understand how implementing social distancing behind bars requires a comprehensive review of workflows and movement; these are eating, accessing medications, and sleeping. Eating behind bars may occur in a centralized dining hall, at tables inside a housing area, or inside an individual cell. Each of these variations involves different approaches to how people get a tray of food and sit to eat, as well as differences in how the food is prepared and delivered. One relatively quick way for facilities to start social distancing during the pandemic was to mark off half the seats in dining areas. This created more distance between people as they ate but increased wait time. It also required more work to keep people spaced out in line or meant adding staff to coordinate smaller groups going to each meal. These problems were often addressed by having meals delivered to the housing areas, and people ate either in their cells or in a common space. These efforts helped keep groups of people in different housing areas from mixing but created a new problem around how and where people would eat, since most housing areas lack sufficient seating for everyone to eat at once, let alone with a space between people. Alternatively, each meal could be served in two shifts, but that resulted in some people getting cold food trays. The success of every one of these permutations relied on the correctional staff being trained and managed to promote distancing. The facilities I inspected where social distancing was working well during meals were the ones that made a commitment to this new role for officers. On the preparation side, several facilities I inspected had outbreaks occur among food workers, either those who worked in the kitchen or those who brought food trays out to housing areas. Key interventions that would have prevented these outbreaks include screening each of these workers for elevated temperature and COVID-19 symptoms before their shifts start and periodically testing them.

One social-distancing challenge that usually went ignored during outbreaks I investigated was the medication line. Behind bars, people usually line up for their medications every day at a cart or window; if there's a program to allow people to keep some medications with them, though, they may line up only every week or two. Either way, there are lines in almost every housing area every day for medications, and the people with the most health problems are in those lines. Almost never would staff or facility administrators come up with a way to keep people spread out in these lines. Because the nurses who hand out the medications are going from one area to another, this is usually a very rushed process. In the few facilities that made changes to medication lines, one person at a time was usually called for their medications, and security and health staff reminded people not to bunch up if there was a line. These seem like common-sense changes, but it takes more time and energy to administer medications this way. And often, without support and monitoring by supervisors, the pressure to get medication carts to multiple housing areas and the demands of other tasks make these changes short-lived.

A final area where social distancing can be implemented but requires ongoing efforts by staff is the sleeping arrangements. Most carceral settings are simply too crowded for a person to maintain six feet or even three feet of distance from others, and some of the most tightly packed spaces are open-bay dorms, where single beds or even bunk beds are lined up two or three feet apart. This crowding is the natural result of mass incarceration, which crams more and more people into spaces designed for fewer. While many of the crowded facilities I've inspected were old and dilapidated, it's important to understand crowding also occurs in newer facilities. In the federal prison in Danbury, Connecticut, the women were held in a relatively new facility that appeared to be a large open warehouse that had been filled with hundreds of bunks, with three-foot-high office-cubicle walls in between smaller groups of bunks. As I reported after my inspection, COVID-19 ripped through this building, and the women were left largely on their own, caring for each other until some of them became gravely ill. Not surprisingly, in open dorms, transmission can be rapid. In addition, these settings reflect the false dichotomy between a locked segregation unit and an open dorm, ignoring other options. The fact is, some units in jails and prisons function well when people have their own cell or room, and they retain the autonomy to come and go without their cell door being locked all day. This approach is common to a small set of units, but it should be standard, as a means to both reduce transmission during outbreaks and improve overall conditions. Of course, housing like this, which is common in European facilities, cannot exist when so many people are being incarcerated and there is a need to warehouse them all.

Most facilities I inspected during COVID-19 took some steps to implement social distancing, and the differences in the effectiveness of these efforts are vast. Some facilities simply ignored the issue of social distancing completely and took the position that, because people in a given housing area were part of the same group or cohort, there wasn't any risk of

COVID-19 spreading. This ignores the reality that COVID-19 was coming in with staff, and that social distancing was about protecting detained people and staff once the virus had arrived with a staff person. Probably the most common approach was to post signs and put tape markings on floors, tables, and chairs to show people how far apart they needed to be. When this was the only approach, these markings and signs were quickly meaningless because there was no actual effort to change the well-established, complicated workflows and patterns. The role of security staff in implementing social distancing was often ignored. Security staff already tell people where to stand, how and when they can congregate, when people can leave their cells or sleeping areas, and when they have to assemble for count three times a day. From the moment a person enters the jail or prison intake, they receive constant orders in this regard. In tightly packed settings like the ones I inspected in the state prisons in Mississippi, there really is no prospect for social distancing.[8] But in many other cases, like the county jails and ICE detention facilities I inspected where the population was closer to 50% of capacity, people were able to distance more effectively—and much more than in those facilities where the security staff just sat back and let people fend for themselves. In the better settings, there was clearly training of correctional staff and real discussion with detained people about distancing. Plus, efforts were made to spread people out for sleeping and other activities like recreation, TV, and meals.

But from the standpoint of public health, not all overcrowding is equally harmful, and even settings that are at 50% capacity can crowd people together in a way that increases health problems. One of the most serious consequences of overcrowding can be violence, especially in cells that hold two to four people but were originally designed for one person. Jailers may place two or more people in the same 8-by-10-foot cell in new admission housing, solitary confinement, and other housing areas with little or no regard for the safety of the people held there. In one such case a man reported that he and his cellmate started to fight almost as soon as the door to their solitary cell was shut, leading to a struggle for survival that included punches, strangling, and wrapping shoelaces and bedsheets around the neck of the other. In the end, one man was dead and the other charged with murder. As psychologist Dr. Craig Haney has said, "We've done this utterly bizarre thing, which is to put two people in cells that were built for one and leave them both in there for 23 or more hours a day."[9]

Eliminating solitary confinement, and especially the practice of double celling people in this setting, is important for violence reduction. But this change also helps to reduce disease transmission between people. Spending 23 or 24 hours per day in a cell with another person virtually ensures any disease that can be transmitted by breathing the same air or by skin-to-skin contact will be. In Florida, where I was part of a team that investigated solitary-confinement conditions, people reported that their property, clothes, and mattresses were taken away by prison guards for perceived slights or disagreements, so they were left in only their underwear for days at a time, sleeping on the floor. They also reported that the supposed daily nurse rounds to detect new health problems were often nonexistent and that correctional officers yelled and threatened them if they tried to get the attention of a passing nurse.[10] Add a new fever, rash, cough, or diarrhea, and the likelihood that a cellmate will not only contract the infection but also deteriorate without care is much higher in a solitary setting. For any outsider coming to help with an outbreak response, it's crucial to examine the special ways solitary can drive transmission and create barriers to diagnosis and treatment.

Another example of how overcrowding can occur when the facility is "under capacity" is the facility intake area. Here, a series of large cells or pens with a single shared toilet and sink usually holds 5–15 people as they pass in and out of the jail or prison. In these pens, people are crammed together so closely they are touching; they sleep on the floor like cordwood and have little or no time out of the pens. Facilities will state that people are only held in these pens for a few hours, but in times of facility crisis, like an outbreak, people may spend days in these settings. In addition, because these pens may inadvertently hold both people who are newly admitted and those who have been in the facility for weeks or months, they are a key way for infections to multiply and spread throughout a facility.

While overcrowding and infection control have been long-standing issues in jails, these failures rapidly accelerated COVID-19 transmission when people were bunched together in intake pens for days at a time. In the New York City jail system, where I previously led the health service, and where we operated under a long-standing mandate to get people through the intake process in 24 hours or less, things fell apart during COVID-19, causing days-long confinement in the intake pens. Dr. Bobby Cohen, a physician who has both led and worked in oversight of this health system, reported that "there were 100-plus people crowded into pens without basic, basic services. Filthy pens without capacity to urinate in a urinal."[11]

I have seen other facilities where the intake area worked in a one-direction manner; meaning, these pens were used only for new people coming in, not for the daily mix of people who leave for court or are released. This approach not only limited the hours people spent in these areas, where transmission could occur, but it also made the job of correctional staff to track the time people had spent in the pens much clearer. On the other end of the spectrum, some facilities use these pens for many reasons aside from intake to the facility, including as housing after a use-of-force incident or during a mental-health emergency. These uses usually occur because the intake area has 24/7 correctional-officer staffing, but the result can be chaos.

Some of the places I've inspected have clearly taken efforts to reduce the number of people in each intake pen and the time spent in these settings to an hour or two; they've also taken efforts to have them cleaned in between uses. Most facilities would state this as standard practice, but by reviewing video and speaking with detained people and staff, it's fairly easy to establish the truth of these facility operations.

In addition to the increased transmission risk that comes with overcrowding in these spaces, the misery, discomfort, and pain associated with them results in people doing what they can to minimize being put there if possible. This is true beyond the intake pens and often includes locked cells that are given a health-related label such as "mental-health watch" and "medical observation." One of the most enduring lessons from COVID-19 has been that using solitary-confinement units for medical isolation creates a strong disincentive for people to report symptoms or seek care. One of the first inspections I conducted was at a federal prison in Manhattan, now closed after multiple problems with almost every part of care, custody, and control. There, a woman reported to me that she was put into the solitary unit, called the SHU, when she became ill:

The first few nights I was in SHU, I had no sheets or blanket. Cold air was blowing out of the vents right over my head on the bed. I think the staff had not been properly educated about COVID-19 at that point because various staff members would walk by me in SHU and make comments like, "Let's see who's infected." I asked the officers for water but they didn't give me any. They told me to just drink from the sink in the cell. I was so dehydrated. One day I was so dehydrated my lips were bleeding and blood was coming through my mask. The medicine they gave me said to take it with a full glass of water. The sink in SHU is full of spit—it is very dirty. I wasn't given cleaning products until about the eighth day I was locked in there, when I was given products and 20 minutes extra to clean the cell. The first two days I was in SHU were the weekend, and no one checked on me. Staff just put food through my door.[12]

This experience would remain the norm for many people in jails and prisons throughout the pandemic. The consequences went beyond suffering in dirty cells without bedding, phone access, reading materials, or their property; it also meant people were quickly reluctant to report symptoms of disease for fear of being punished with these conditions. The need to eliminate this punitive approach was part of my assessment of the federal prison in Lompoc, California, and coming to grips with the punitive approach to medical isolation has been a serious problem throughout many of the inspections I've conducted.[13]

But I've also evaluated places where staff have listened to people's complaints about how degrading and unsafe these settings are, and they have developed more humane and clinically appropriate medical isolation. In the women's prison

in Virginia, called Fluvanna, the facility staff used a cell housing area for medical isolation, but they made the critical decision that people didn't need to have the doors of their cells
locked during the daytime hours, allowing them to come and
go from the common area outside the cells. This was possible
because the unit was not being used at the time for solitary
confinement or another security-related reason. It was also
possible because the health staff recognized that once people
tested positive, it was fine for them to be in a housing area with
other positive people—and that there was no health benefit to
keeping people locked in small cells 24/7. In the Lompoc facility, where I'd reported repeatedly on the harms of using the
SHU for medical isolation, staff did eventually develop alternative approaches. In one building they used a mothballed
housing area for people who tested positive, and they took the
same approach as Fluvanna, not locking people into the cells
and allowing them phone calls and access to their property.
This approach to medical isolation is important because it
works to remove the punishing elements of segregation or solitary units that drive people to keep their symptoms hidden.
When I asked people at Lompoc and other jails, prisons, and
detention centers about why they were reluctant to report
COVID-19 symptoms, not wanting to be transferred to a punitive setting was the most common response. This is an area
where the CDC's guidelines were somewhat helpful. About
six months into the COVID-19 pandemic, the CDC added
language to their detention guidelines saying that medical
isolation should not be punitive, but they didn't explicitly state
that solitary units shouldn't be used for medical isolation, especially when both functions were being conducted.[14] As with
the CDC's lack of clear language on release, this ambiguity
let facilities assume that if they made some efforts to make

solitary somehow more hospitable, then placing people with COVID-19 into active solitary units would be allowable.

Aside from limiting how many people are in a facility during an outbreak, another important tool for saving lives is to screen staff and detained people for symptoms. Screening involves actively looking for new symptoms, both by asking questions and by taking temperatures, or using other objective means. This active effort is different from simply waiting for people to recognize and report their symptoms and is needed to catch infections early and initiate treatment, as well as to reduce transmission from one person to another. We used daily screenings during a legionella outbreak at Rikers when I was part of Correctional Health Services. We knew infections were localized to one or two facilities, and we were especially worried about a subset of high-risk patients. The CDC identified this as essential during the COVID-19 pandemic as well, making clear that staff and any detained people who were in quarantine should be screened on a daily basis.[15] While many of the facilities I inspected failed to do this, some took it seriously and were able to catch infections early. At the Bureau of Prisons facility at Lompoc, the leadership used a separate building for every security and civilian staff member to pass through on the way to their shift. One of the impressive features about this screening was that it had a pathway clearly marked and separated, so that people would enter one door, follow a line to a first station, then proceed to a second station, all while maintaining social distancing. In general, the spread-out nature of most rural prisons and county jails made this type of setup much more possible. In urban facilities, the staff often enter one door, and several feet away they clear the magnetometer and other security processes. Wedging a COVID-19 questionnaire and temperature check into this area was difficult in many of the settings I observed, and some elected instead to employ a second office or entrance as a COVID-19 screening site.

One other helpful response to COVID-19 was the elimination of co-pays for health care. In many detention settings, people must pay a charge, often $3–7 for access to care using the sick-call system. Patients have long described to me how this charge limits their ability to receive care. In theory, there are avenues for indigent people to receive care without a charge, and also in theory, these charges are waived for certain urgent or emergent scenarios. In reality, the social-services staff who assist with indigent services are often unavailable. And when co-pays are charged to patients incorrectly, they must endure a long and often unsuccessful appeal process that can bring retaliation or even less care. In addition, these co-pays are often for gateway care, such as nurse triage, which must be accessed two or three times before a person can see a physician, thus requiring multiple charges. When COVID-19 started in early 2020, most correctional settings with co-pays tried to communicate that COVID-19-related co-pays would be suspended. But my early inspections in 2020 revealed people were still being charged for seeking care directly related to COVID-19, which in some settings created a disincentive to reporting new symptoms. This confusion led a number of facilities to do away with their co-pays altogether—a move that some facilities have maintained, without being overwhelmed by new demand.

There are many other interventions that work well to reduce transmission, morbidity, and mortality during outbreaks. Some of the innovations I've encountered are daily screening of work crews, use of biodegradable laundry bags, and standardized training for cleaning crews, whether staffed by security or detained people. Some of the easiest and most important interventions revolve around the facility-intake areas. As mentioned earlier, some of them can be reworked to become one-way, only used for people arriving from the outside. Having PPE, reliable cleaning, and access to bathrooms and showers in these places seems pretty basic but is hard to maintain because they are so busy, often unpredictably so. Having PPE, cleaning, and sanitation for transport vehicles and staff also seems rudimentary but is hard to maintain when there isn't a clear infection-control officer on the security side. Other responses, like reducing admissions and interfacility transfers, building new onsite hospitals, or procuring medical isolation rooms in prefab containers, require significant funding and outside coordination.

While most of the discussion in this chapter is about what works to reduce morbidity and mortality, it's important to keep an eye on another driving force behind bars: financial profit. I encountered this issue when considering air-quality improvements. It's not hard to imagine how bad the air quality is behind bars and the ways this can drive outbreaks of airborne infections. Inside a locked cell, inside a housing area, and throughout the congregate areas like day rooms, hallways, clinics, and program spaces, there is almost no tracking or effort to improve air quality during outbreaks. The two important variables in air quality are ventilation and filtration, with the first referring to the exchange of inside air with outside air, and the second referring to the cleaning of the air, usually through filters that trap or remove specific viral and other kinds of particles.[16] I raise this because when COVID-19 arrived, we already knew plenty of well-evidenced ways to improve both ventilation and filtration. For prison systems that wanted to prevent the spread of COVID-19, they could improve these parts of the physical facility, but they could also spend money to hire infection-control staff, ensure adequate nursing staff were present, and follow CDC recommendations to limit morbidity and mortality. In Arkansas state prisons, the decision was made to deploy $2 million worth of air ionizers in housing areas. I was critical of this move in my COVID-19 inspection report, noting that while these tools had been tested in a lab, they had not yet been proven in conditions like an open dorm, where the device was in a duct 15 feet above the closely stacked beds and where social distancing and basic COVID-19 testing hadn't been implemented. I also reported that

> Boeing, for example, considered installing these types of devices on their passenger planes, but declined to do so after independent testing. Although air-purification devices may bring some benefits in housing areas where people reside in individual rooms, it is unlikely that they could have a meaningful impact on transmission from one person to another in the many open dorms where beds are placed 2 feet apart or less. In these dorm areas, people are arranged in cramped quarters along a long narrow open area and the ionizing device is inside an air duct 13–15 feet above them, with little air movement down at the level where people sit and sleep (Ex. 7 IMG DSCN 2199). There was no effort to space these bunks farther apart because of COVID-19 or to keep every other bunk empty, both of which I have observed as basic COVID-19 social distancing measures in jails and prisons since early 2020.[17]

The creep of graft and profit motives into mass incarceration is nothing new, but every new crisis can weaken already feeble oversight and accountability mechanisms. My experience is, left unchecked, the money intended for basic services and care behind bars is quickly diverted toward contracts that bring profit to some without helping incarcerated people or staff. One of the best detailed accounts of the scope of potential kickbacks in a system was reported by the *Clarion Ledger* in Mississippi and revealed years of kickbacks involving the top officials of the state prison system, ranging from phone to facility contracts.[18] In Nassau County, New York, the graft in the county executive's office involved hundreds of thousands of dollars in contracts between the jail and a local bakery being paid to provide bread and rolls.[19] Even when the law isn't being broken, the gouging of incarcerated people and their families with expensive phone contracts and overpriced access to tablets and other tech devices represents a core area of profits for large corporations.[20] Recent lawsuits have alleged that not only do the phone-service companies fix prices but that they may give kickbacks to facilities for agreeing to cut in-person visits.[21]

Finally, a key tool we need to save lives during an outbreak is for health departments and the CDC to be involved in providing specific guidance and feedback to facilities. This means going into facilities, evaluating the timing and adequacy of the facility responses, and being honest about deficiencies and how practices may be harming health. In the facilities where I saw this in practice, the health agency already had a relationship with the prison or jail based on work that was in place before the outbreak, and their staff already had been visiting the facility, meeting confidentially with incarcerated people, and helping the facility do better. If this type of relationship isn't established before an outbreak, it's more likely that when outside public-health staffers arrive in response to an outbreak, they will end up receiving nothing more than a guided tour from the facility administrators. Even if they do speak to incarcerated people, these meetings can be curated to exclude those who are critical of how things are going. Arranging confidential interviews with incarcerated people and health staff can greatly assist in learning about gaps in facility resources and policies.

One of the most compelling parts of walking into a facility during an outbreak is seeing how extremely stressed and overworked the staff and leaders are, and it is usually clear they have undertaken numerous steps to mitigate the effects of the outbreak. Because these people are usually the main contacts that outside public-health investigators have when doing an assessment, in a very human response, investigators tend to appreciate those staff for their efforts and sacrifices and to give suggestions about how to improve things in a way that doesn't disrespect their work. But if the same outside team met confidentially with incarcerated people, they might get a completely different story about an outbreak. They might hear that the facility had ignored cases and had responded to health symptoms with abuse or neglect, and that people behind bars were caring for each other because they couldn't get any other help. If the staff and incarcerated people offer completely different takes on some key parts of the outbreak response, then video footage, medical records, security logs, and other data sources could be used to help the outside health agency sort out reality. But many external reviews of outbreak response stop after the first step, and investigators see and hear only what the facility staff want them to consider. The consequence isn't just that they fail to get to the truth of the outbreak. By learning and reporting the efforts of the staff in the facility and ignoring the experience of the people detained there, outside health staffers take part in dehumanizing incarcerated people; they see and hear one perspective and not another. This cycle, which plays out in a thousand other ways before and after these outside health staff arrive, is a crucially toxic one, because it brings the credibility of the outside health agency to bear in the worst way. When a sheriff or correctional leader touts the great job they've done and cites the endorsement of a health department as evidence, even if the assessment was this type of one-sided affair, the health department or agency has given their seal of approval. But they've also sent a clear message to the people locked up in that facility: we don't believe you and don't need to consider your viewpoint.

So maybe the most essential tool for facilities is one they all have access to already, and that's engaging with detained people about what is happening. I know that detained people aren't usually asked about quality or access to health care before a crisis, so the idea that a MRSA, scabies, or COVID-19 outbreak will trigger engagement can seem far-fetched. But for an outside public-health staffer, the opportunity exists to take this approach. This kind of outsider has a unique opportunity to consider the divide in perspectives, if one exists, on what is really happening in the facility. Each group—health staff, security staff, and patients—have different experiences, and each can easily have a different impression of reality, without any malice or ill-intent. Finding ways to understand and communicate these issues is a responsibility an outside public-health staffer is uniquely prepared to tackle, and the benefits of doing so include a better outbreak response and the opportunity to improve the health system.

Recommendations

- Consider release and diversion from incarceration of high-risk people.

- Create increased protections for high-risk people, including cohorting in special housing areas with increased infection control and clinical surveillance.
- Use the full space of the facility to ensure social distancing in housing areas.
- Engage local and state health departments for guidance on outbreak responses, and follow up with public reporting of findings and corrective actions and recommendations.
- Avoid use of solitary confinement and intake areas for medical isolation. Ensure that medical isolation is nonpunitive and includes access to phone, recreation, property, and commissary.
- Eliminate co-pays for health services.

Research ideas
- Hypothesis: Release of older and other medically vulnerable people can be implemented as part of outbreak response in a way that promotes public safety. Approach: Review recent efforts to promote release as a public-health tool.[22] Review lawsuits that may provide information in this area.[23]
- Hypothesis: Elimination of co-pays during COVID-19 did not create any financial burdens, nor did it result in overwhelming correctional health services with sick-call and other care requests. Approach: Examine the natural experiment that occurs when co-pays are suspended or eliminated to detect how the number of requests for care or the administrative work to process co-pays is impacted.

APPENDIX

A Practical Guide to Inspecting a Jail
or Prison Outbreak

This chapter is intended as a resource for public-health staffers conducting a visit or inspection of a facility regarding a communicable-disease outbreak. This guide offers recommendations on the path of the inspection, including the approach to interviews and how to scale the inspection based on the extent of the outbreak and size of the facility.

Whatever physical places you see on your visit, remember the facility leaders are showing you what they want you to see. Some of their team may be genuinely looking for help, while others may be simply seeking a stamp of approval to show any efforts they've made are adequate.[1] There has likely been considerable cleaning, moving of people, and extra staffing allocated to make whatever you see today quite different from what existed yesterday or the day before.

The inspection will not yield credible impressions about the outbreak without confidential interviews with detained people. Your physical inspection is important, just like the opinions of staff and other information.[2] But if you do not confidentially ask people impacted by the outbreak about their experience, then you have missed the most granular details about what works and what needs fixing.

Inspection path. Below are the steps and considerations for most inspections, followed by a few details on each area that might relate to outbreaks.

- Welcome or sit-down meeting
- Intake and receiving areas
- New admission or classification housing areas
- Medical clinic and infirmary
- Mental-health, geriatric, and disability housing areas

- General population housing areas, male and female
- Restrictive housing areas and segregation
- Places people work, including kitchen and laundry areas
- Affected housing areas—where the outbreak is occurring
- Confidential interviews
- Considering the scale of the investigation
- Readout meeting

Welcome or sit-down meeting. This is usually the first step of the day and occurs in the warden or sheriff's conference room. Try to keep this meeting as short as possible. It should focus on the path of the inspection and the rules and protocols for the day. You will want to dig in to the status of the outbreak, get a list of cases and potential exposures, and hear about the screening, testing, diagnosis, and treatment efforts. Try to get as much of this information as possible in the days before your visit by phone or video meeting so you can receive just a brief update when you arrive. If you have a team of more than one or two people and are pressed for time, you could have someone stick with the facility leadership to take a closer look at these details while others conduct the inspection.

Some important questions to settle before you start the inspection include the following:[3]

- Can you have brief chats with either staff or detained people in the areas you pass through?[4]
- Can you take pictures or have the security staff take pictures at your direction?
- How much time do you have, including breaks, and where will any confidential interviews occur?
- Do the outbreak responses in screening, testing, or treatment differ for staff and detained people?
- Can you see current mitigation efforts in action?
- Are there housing areas for medical, mental-health, substance-use, and other concerns?[5]

Intake and receiving areas. See the intake cells or pens, and ask about their function. This could include housing people who are newly arrested, those going to and returning from court or medical visits, and people on their way out for release or other reasons. Try to ask about how long people spend in these cells; in some places it may be two to six hours, and in others it may be days. See where toilets and sinks are located for people in the intake areas, including people in isolation cells.[6] See and ask about the maximum number of people in each pen or cell. Lots of transmission occurs in these cells during outbreaks, and any thoughts about keeping people separated based on outbreak status may not actually hold true here. Ask about how contact tracing is done for exposures among detained people and staff who are in this area.

See where the initial health screening and other encounters with health staff occur in this area. Consider whether questions that relate to the outbreak are asked in a confidential setting or in a place where other detained people and correctional officers (COs) can hear responses. Determine whether cells are used for any kind of intoxication, withdrawal, or mental-health crisis, and whether a person going into one of these cells stops getting basic screening, diagnosis, and treatment for infection.

New admission or classification housing areas. This is a set of housing areas where people go in their first week or two of detention. These types of units can serve security functions to figure out different classification levels (like minimum, medium, or maximum custody) or to carry out medical requirements, so that TB, COVID-19, or other initial screening can occur. During an outbreak, these units allow for more screening to occur.

If these areas do exist, one common issue with them is the constant flow in and out of each unit. They are good for screening and testing individuals, but without a rigorous method of batching people together, they don't usually stop the spread of communicable infection to other areas. If people are locked into cells for this phase, then their interaction with others and transmission will be limited, but this is very punitive and isolating, and it risks people being ill without being able to report it or receive treatment.

You might find it helpful to announce yourself to the unit and tell people that they aren't required to speak with you but that you can have brief chats with them about the outbreak. You should then walk through the units to see cells or dorms, bathrooms, recreation areas, and common areas.[7]

In any housing area, see how people get sick-call forms or request care. Ask to see the forms and get a copy. If the requests are done at a kiosk, ask to see it, and ask a person on the unit to show you their requests and responses on the kiosk without security looking over your shoulder. Ask where people who live on that unit are seen for sick call and where the COs are stationed on the unit, especially at night and on weekends. Ask about access to care for emergencies, including how long it takes to get COs and medical staff to the housing area, again especially at night and on weekends. In addition, ask whether people have access to soap and paper towels in the bathroom, and check for yourself. Take photos of the bathroom, including showers, and note the number of showers, sinks, and toilets that are not working on the unit. Go inside and photograph at least one cell per housing area; look for and photograph loose trash and food trays on the floor. Speak with at least one person who cleans the unit.[8]

Medical clinic and infirmary. In the clinic, ask to see patient-care areas, where cultures or other diagnostic procedures happen, and supplies used. Ask whether there is 24/7 nursing staff and what the hours are for physician and mid-level-care providers.[9] If there is an infirmary, see how many open dorms compared to cells or rooms there are and how isolated people and people with infection are kept separate from others. Ask how they shower, use the phone, and are provided meals. Observe whether relevant signage is present for the appropriate precaution levels, and ask health and security staff what it means. Also ask patients when those signs were posted. Try to detect differences in infection-control measures for men's and women's clinic and infirmary areas. Assess whether people in an infirmary setting can call for help; test their call bells or buzzers; ask them about response time and their care overall. Because infirmary patients may not be able to move, it often makes sense to do a few of these interviews as you pass through, which can take an hour or so. If people are in medical isolation, you can save those interviews for the end of the inspection.

Mental-health, geriatric, and disability housing areas. People with a health issue are placed in these areas, but these patients may not get an appropriate level of infection control or health-care access. The same questions asked about new admission housing are relevant here, but it's also important to detect barriers between a person and the sick-call form, the sick-call nurse, and medications. These barriers might occur because people in these units spend most or all of their day in a locked cell. Or they may lack the physical ability to walk far enough to seek care, or they may not hear or see that sick call or other health activities are happening. If medication nurses who pass by are the ones who provide and collect the sick-call forms, ask about whether they always carry forms and always accept them. In ADA-related housing, check for shared wheelchairs, showers, and other assistive devices or accommodations.

General population housing areas. Ask the same questions you would ask in new admission housing areas. Seeing male and female housing is especially important.

Restrictive housing areas and segregation. These areas include disciplinary and administrative segregation; meaning, they contain people who are being punished for violating a facility rule (disciplinary) and those the facility thinks are dangerous, as well as those who haven't been given a rules infraction (administrative). These areas also include protective custody and any housing areas for 17-year-olds and for LGBTQ+ people—all of which can be run just like punishment units, with people held for 23 or more hours a day in locked cells. Key things to figure out are access to sick-call forms, nursing care, and which of these areas has some form of informal or off-the-books punishment. This is often a cell or unit where security staff may put someone for punishment, but not give them an infraction or hearing, and then send them back to their regular housing. Because it's informal, medical staff may miss this kind of transfer and lose track of people who are cases or exposed to cases of the outbreak. It's important to make sure people haven't been recently moved into these areas to hide cases of infection or to silence people reporting parts of the outbreak. Ask the same questions about how people get sick-call forms and are seen, since people can have outbreak symptoms that are ignored for days or weeks in these settings.

Places people work, including kitchen and laundry areas. This is a broad set of possible physical spaces and work settings, so the key is to map out what jobs are done by incarcerated people, how they get to and from work, and where they live. Some facilities have dedicated work crews that live in selected housing areas. Also, it's important to see whether the facility has any screening for health status before each shift. Speak with some of these workers and ask what happens when they are sick. The facility will likely provide a policy or protocol stating a CO supervises these workers, and claiming that, whenever someone reports feeling ill, they are sent for medical care or don't work.[10]

Affected housing areas—where the outbreak is occurring. I usually make this the last spot to visit so that any higher-level PPE and infection-control measures can be held off until the end. For people with acute infection, it's important to ask about and see how they receive routine care and how they call for assistance. Test the call bells or duress alarms. Also, see where the nearest examination space is. If there's a sick-call room or office in the same space, then nursing or medical staff can evaluate a patient without leaving the area. If there isn't, and if there is any risk of transmission to others, then it's a lot less likely the person is really taken off the unit for care very often, and most of the "assessments" are likely made cell side or without a real physical exam. Make sure to seek out and speak with people who are recorded as "recovered."

Confidential interviews. An essential part of any inspection is holding confidential interviews with incarcerated people and, if possible, staff. Depending on how you came to be in the facility (lawsuit or monitoring or invitation), some of these interviews may be difficult to get agreement on. On the day of a visit, I would always prioritize the interviews with detained people over the ones with staff; you can do a phone or video interview with staff afterward. The basic parts of these interviews involve questions about the outbreak, general questions about the health and security services that bear on the outbreak, and at least one question about threats or intimidation regarding speaking with you. Selecting who to speak with should be driven by your walk-through and health priorities. So, if the facility provides people for you to interview, make sure to also find some people on your own to compare experiences.

There may be a couple of basic questions you ask in each chat that contribute to overall information gathering. These chats may yield many interested people, so the goal at this stage is usually to keep each chat short, focus on questions relevant to the outbreak and related health services, and identify people who seem to have important information to share and from whom you can take their name and number and see confidentially later.

Most discussions fall into two types: brief chats in housing areas or in-depth interviews in a confidential room. But sometimes there may be a mixture of the two. For example, if a lot of people want to speak in a housing area, you can take a table in the day room and speak with people one at a time, after asking security to stay back out of earshot. In the infirmary, it might be a challenge to move anywhere else to speak, so having longer discussions right at a person's bedside can work well. Interviews behind bars can be confidential in terms of what you are told, but it's not possible to keep the identity of the person speaking to you from security staff.

There is usually some clinical leadership present at the welcome meeting in the morning and during the inspection that you might think you want to interview, such as a sick-call nurse or infection-control officer. If any staff interviews are possible, the facility may offer the health services administrator. This person usually runs the health service and is most knowledgeable about the scope of services and the intersection between health and security services. In for-profit models of care, this person is also the one corporate HQ relies on to minimize fines and complaints, and to keep the contract partner (the sheriff or corrections department) happy. The directors of nursing and medicine have more purely clinical roles. Their take on challenges to the implementation of outbreak responses are important but may be overshadowed by the health services administrator.

Considering the scale of the investigation. For smaller outbreaks, like a handful of MRSA cases, it may make sense to see just the intake and receiving area, the medical clinic or infirmary, and the housing areas where people with the infection were or are located. Think about who could be missed by current methods; for example, for skin-infection outbreaks, ask for all sick-call and grievance forms relating to a lesion, boil, or ulcer as a possible denominator. Gathering more granular detail on the total number of cases of skin ulcers reported by sick call compared to the number of cases that got a culture done, and what happened after, is important. How and where each of those steps occurred should be examined, including lab pickup and the review and documentation of results. Also consider whether discharge planning is relevant.[11]

For outbreaks that involve multiple areas, or in situations where widespread transmission is possible, it is important to see much more of the facility than usual, since movement of staff and detained people through the entire facility is crucial for proposing mitigation steps. A scalable approach to interviews is also possible. If there are only a handful of cases, interviewing those people and a few more people in their housing areas could suffice; meaning, 5–10 people are interviewed. For a more widespread concern, it's important to interview men and women, those with serious preexisting health problems, and those in general population, segregation, and medical and mental-health housing units; meaning, 15–30 people may be the goal. In most of my inspections, I would speak with 10–15 people on a one-day visit, 30 or so if I had two days, and up to 75 if I had three or four days. Those interactions would be a mix of shorter 2–5-minute chats and a smaller number of longer interviews, usually 15–45 minutes. If you're stumped on who to speak with, ask the local public defender or protection and advocacy groups before you go. They likely have staff who would love to tell you about the facility beforehand and suggest people to speak with.

Readout meeting. Most of the time, facility leadership wants to get some feedback at the end of the inspection. Even during litigation, this sometimes occurs, but it is more expected when a health-department team has been invited. It is very important to not give feedback that can be interpreted as your conclusions or findings—it's usually necessary to review more information before this can occur. Using terms like "first impressions" can help keep your feedback grounded. Make sure to thank the staff who escorted you and made the inspection possible. It's likely that a lot of work was pushed aside to make the visit happen and still awaits once you leave. It's also important to give feedback on any true emergencies you see, especially those related to fixable risks of morbidity and mortality. Specific concerns about people you spoke with may be important to share with the clinical team if there is an urgent or emergent issue, but be sure to raise them in your interview with the person too. Examples of these concerns include a person not getting a life-sustaining medication or experiencing untreated illness or injury. Also, any staff working behind bars should know about the Prison Rape

Elimination Act (PREA) and their obligations to report sexual abuse.[12]

Final Thoughts

After many years conducting inspections and investigations behind bars, I've come to one basic premise about uncovering the truth in these situations. *The real detective work is not determining the disease epidemiology—it's finding the people missing from a denominator.* By that I mean, who reported symptoms that never got assessed? Who is considered recovered but is still acutely ill? Who are the high-risk patients? You should seek sick-call forms and medical grievances over a time frame you select to help answer these questions, but—as I've stressed before—holding confidential interviews with patients is essential.

If the information above makes sense, *take action*! When outside public-health staff visit a jail or prison, their efforts often end with accepting the facility narrative about an outbreak and offering support or congratulations for all the hard work. Taking action means following up on data questions or concerns that were brushed aside or not addressed, like infection-control staffing, line lists of cases or documentation surveillance, and contact tracing. One area that is often unclear relates to roles in screening, surveillance, and care—who does each of the specific tasks the facility has put in place? And who does these tasks overnight and on weekends when staffing is much lower? During your visit, other people in the room may not want to cause any annoyance—or they may actively want you to take home the perspectives of facility staff. Even if they aren't hiding anything, facility leadership have very different information than detained people have.

Once you've visited a facility, find a way to tell other people about what you've learned. And keep finding more ways to go back. So few public-health professionals ever visit these settings (there are approximately 7,000 jails, prisons, and detention centers in the United States) that we need to get your insights and thoughts to add to a wider perspective of public health. One opportunity is to provide support or training in infection control to correctional officers.[13] Think about how your organization could have a more substantial connection to this facility over time, and how you might get information about other public-health issues from incarcerated people and staff.

Finally, think about how hiring someone who has been incarcerated can help your work. People who have been held in a jail, prison, or detention center have a far deeper understanding of health risks and services, and their knowledge is vital for your other team members. This is doubly true for finding and interpreting data once an index case and some spread of disease has occurred. The ways close contact occurs and can be monitored isn't always clear, but people who have lived experience of incarceration will have navigated some of the same hallways, clinics, and housing areas, and they can greatly benefit any team investigating an outbreak.

Notes

1. It's important to know how different the standards of care are in carceral spaces. Because most state health departments, the Centers for Medicare and Medicaid Services, and other public-health structures are usually not part of delivery or oversight of care, incarcerated people often need to show deliberate indifference in their care to get a sanction against a facility in a lawsuit, which requires meeting a far higher bar than simply showing they don't get evidence-based care or the standard of care. For more, see the ACLU's Know Your Rights resource at https://www.aclu.org/sites/default/files/images/asset_upload_file690_25743.pdf.

2. Other important data sources include sick-call forms, medical grievances, medical records of affected people, video footage, and administrative documents like staffing and housing-area records. A couple of important staffing issues to learn about are the number of unfilled nurse and correctional-officer

positions as well as whether there are dedicated infection-control staff. I've often learned that a facility has a full-time infection-control nurse designated on their staffing matrix but the position is unfilled, and this title and critical work has simply been assigned to another nurse with other full-time responsibilities.

3. Here are some further logistics to consider: A laptop will help with the sit-down part of the inspection, but it might not be allowed in the main facility. You will most likely need a small five-by-eight or similar notebook to use in the housing areas. Tablet computers work fine once you have a template for inspection, but I was always more efficient in the brief chats with a pen and paper notebook. I'm a fan of cargo pants—they let you carry some extra PPE, and they can hold your notebook and pens so you can walk around with your hands free. The stairs and floors of housing areas are often covered with trip-and-fall hazards, so watch where you step. If you'll do more than one of these visits, consider buying a clear plastic tote bag for your computer and snacks. Some state prisons have rules about not bringing cash into the facility, so be prepared to bring just your ID. Some medium- and high-security prisons require you to wear a tactical vest, which is for protection from slashing. Also, I have always relied on shoes that slip on and off and that are good for wading in a little water or mud. Even if the housing areas aren't flooded, some prisons require a fair amount of outdoor walking. I always wear a watch during inspections since phones aren't usually allowed and there is a natural tendency to spend a lot of time on the most positive, clean, and prepared parts of the facility, and it's important to make time to get to the places you think are relevant to the outbreak. For the inspection photos, whether you, your colleagues, or a member of the facility team takes them, consider taking one photo of the entrance door to each unit you see. This gives you an easy record in the photos of where you went, although you will also keep notes about every picture. It's hard to take and log photos while also taking other notes, so having a security person handle the photos

works well—also, they usually need to vet the photos for security issues afterward.

4. These should take two to five minutes, and the goal is to ask a few basic questions and identify people for later confidential interviews. Security staff should stay back six feet or so during these chats. If you aren't allowed to interview staff, ask whether you can talk to staff about specific things you see along the way, such as, "What is this cell for?" and "How do people in this unit get a sick-call form?"

5. Other possibilities include pregnancy, geriatric, and ADA concerns. Ask to see any special groups kept separate from others, including 17-year-olds, ICE detainees, transfers from other systems, and those in protective custody. These people may have much more restrictive placements that hamper infection control and access to care. If the people in these areas are especially vulnerable, ask whether correctional staff is steady (whether there is a smaller group of dedicated staff for each unit).

6. Many intake areas have cells for holding people in active mental-health crisis or being observed for intoxication or withdrawal. This practice can increase morbidity and mortality because it isolates people experiencing complex medical or psychiatric crises and incorrectly supposes that periodically looking through a locked cell door constitutes adequate medical monitoring. It also stops other medical assessments, including screening for the outbreak disease and conducting a close-contact investigation.

7. Making an announcement in the housing area has a few benefits. It lets you size up how people react to you, and it also lets them know you are not one of the facility health staff. If there is a lot of anger regarding being locked down or other facility problems, you may get a quick and hostile response because you're walking in with the facility leadership. It's worth asking the facility staff whether you can answer questions about the outbreak when you announce yourself. This might not feel comfortable because you will get some questions about

access to care, but if you can tell people you're there from the outside and don't work in the facility, you can be a valuable source of information for detained people and COs. You might answer a random question or two, or a much larger opportunity might present itself, like an impromptu town hall where the entire housing area is asking questions. If this happens, see if you can find a way to answer as many questions as possible about the pathology and basics of transmission, because the facility has likely not done this type of education and updating, and people may be completely in the dark. You might also hear people complain about the facility's response. I would tell those people you'd like to talk to them confidentially. But be sure to field some of the more general questions if the facility team allows and if you feel comfortable.

8. Each housing area usually has a few people tasked with cleaning that area. These workers usually get supplies from the housing-area COs and have a view of how the unit works generally and whether conditions the day of inspection reflect what they normally experience.

9. The term "infirmary" usually refers to a place where patients are in 24/7 eyesight and earshot of health staff. This is different from an observation cell, where there isn't constant oversight but rather intermittent correctional or health checks.

10. This is rarely the case in reality; often people face pressure or retaliation for failing to work. Remember, in prison systems, incarcerated people can legally be used as slave labor, and work is often forced. This affects whether people can simply take a day off when they are sick. Also, work not done by incarcerated people may get shifted to COs, like running food trays from the kitchen to the housing areas, or doing basic maintenance, so the pressure to keep people working in their jobs may cut against the stated outbreak-screening measures.

11. The outbreak may create a need to track symptoms or ensure medication continuity when people go home; for example, they may need to take a course of antivirals or antibiotics. If so, ask if

there is a discharge-planning process already established. This process involves people being identified by health staff to come through the clinic or otherwise see a nurse before they go home. This protocol allows health staff to create a flag for security staff, making sure a person goes home with appointments and medications, which can be useful during an outbreak.

12.   PREA is a federal law that establishes basic and mandatory training, prevention, treatment, and documentation standards for sexual abuse in carceral settings. If someone tells you they have been sexually abused, you need to report this to the PREA coordinator or another member of the facility leadership. If you are working with attorneys on your team, this is the type of issue you can report to them so they can interface with the appropriate person or team in the facility, including noting any reports that a PREA issue was ignored. For more information, see https://www.prearesourcecenter.org/standard /115-61.

13.   This has been a great approach in areas like traumatic brain injury, suicide prevention, overdose response, and other concrete subjects where the leadership are keen for any brief training or support that outside groups can give their staff. Also, the employee health office of many jails and prisons is focused on maintaining staffing and may not focus on infection control for their staff.

ACKNOWLEDGMENTS

The motivation for *Outbreak Behind Bars* comes largely from incarcerated people. If you skip to the end of the book, in the appendix you'll find a short field guide of sorts on how to approach a facility visit or inspection. That guide and the preceding chapters emphasize that getting the confidential input of incarcerated people is an absolute requirement when responding to an outbreak.

In service of this principle, I want to acknowledge the over 1,000 incarcerated people I've interviewed in the past several years and to share some examples that show why speaking with incarcerated people is required when responding to an outbreak. Their reports have typically included what is working well in outbreak responses, along with deficiencies; consistency between these reports has been crucial to my understanding of reality.

Jails, prisons, and detention centers operate with extreme disparities in power. It's important to learn about how well or poorly infection-control principles are integrated. In one prison, I toured the dining hall when it wasn't in use and saw that each of the round metal tables had two of the four seats removed, leaving two seats and two thin metal slats where the seats had been. This was presented as a basic social-distancing measure by the facility, but when I counted the number of people who would eat during these half-filled sessions, it was hard to imagine the facility could get everyone fed. When I spoke with people incarcerated at the facility, they said that people still came in pretty much the same number as before but that anyone known as a sex offender was forced to sit on the metal slats, leaving three or four people at a table like before.

In another facility, I learned that on high-heat days, some solitary cells were not air-conditioned and could become extremely hot. As a remedial measure on hot days, the facility reported they would bring in large fans and point them at the cell fronts with a basin of ice directly in front of the fan, to move colder air toward the cells. People in one of these solitary units reported that the facility was consistent about setting up these measures on hot days but that the fans were pointed at the desks of the correctional officers, not the solitary cells.

The actual experiences of incarcerated people are equally important for learning about successful outbreak measures. In one prison, facility administrators told me the inmate work crews were screened every morning as a COVID-19 measure before going to their shifts. I'd heard this in many settings but rarely found it to be true since the job of screening incarcerated people often fell to a correctional officer with many other responsibilities and little incentive to hold people back from work, especially if a lack of workers meant more hassle and work for officers. But when I interviewed incarcerated people on these work crews, I found that not only were they being screened every day but that health staff were doing these screenings and both documenting the interactions and getting people seen right away when they were too sick to work.

In another facility, people I interviewed said that during an outbreak they were allowed to get their medications in a 7- or 30-day supply instead of congregating in line at a medication cart every day for each individual pill. They said this had decreased their close contact with other people and made their medication management easier because they were now in charge of initiating a refill request.

One of the unexpected realities I learned from incarcerated people involved how a successful infection-control measure might be implemented for men but not women. Men held in one facility I inspected reported that, when they arrived, they would spend time in the intake pens, then go to new admission housing, and if anyone had a mental-health emergency after arrival, they would be transferred to a separate mental-health unit.

Women I interviewed reported a different process, which involved being taken back to intake pens for observation during mental-health emergencies because there was no dedicated women's mental-health unit. They gave detailed accounts of how this led to them contracting COVID-19 from newly arrived women held in these same pens. They also gave credible accounts of how this process led to transmission in the rest of the facility when they were cleared from their mental-health emergency and returned to their original housing areas.

An eye-opening part of conducting these interviews around outbreaks has been learning to rethink what really matters in infection control, screening, diagnosis, and treatment behind bars. Staffing of correctional officers is one of these elements. One prison I inspected had such serious staffing shortages that, at certain times, one officer might be "guarding" up to 400 incarcerated people held in numerous housing units. Both the incarcerated people and health staff I interviewed reported serious barriers for a person who was feeling ill to be seen by medical staff because there was often nobody to tell. As a result, there was little practical way to implement the rapid assessment of people with new disease symptoms. In many of the facilities I've inspected, people report having to bang on doors, yell, and even start fires to get the attention of staff for health emergencies. This dynamic of neglect and the need to clamor for care isn't present everywhere, but when it does exist, it can render the facility outbreak-response plan ineffective.

For public-health professionals walking into a jail, prison, or detention center, connecting with incarcerated people and getting their insights will yield far better outcomes for outbreak response and prevention.

NOTES

1. Germs and Jails

1. Much of Mr. Oya's story was reported by University of Utah epidemiologist Dr. Katharine Walter in the *Nation*. Walter KS. Meet Dennis Oya, Patient Zero of the TB Outbreak Sweeping Washington's Prisons. *Nation*. January 30, 2023. https://www .thenation.com/article/society/tb-washington-state-prisons/.

2. Walter. Meet Dennis Oya.

3. Stalter RM, Pecha M, Dov L, et al. Tuberculosis Outbreak in a State Prison System—Washington, 2021–2022. *Morbidity and Mortality Weekly Report*. March 24, 2023. https://www.cdc .gov/mmwr/volumes/72/wr/mm7212a3.htm.

4. Clinical Overview of Latent Tuberculosis Infection. Centers for Disease Control and Prevention. May 8, 2024. https://www .cdc.gov/tb/hcp/clinical-overview/latent-tuberculosis -infection.html?CDC_AAref_Val=https://www.cdc.gov/tb /publications/factsheets/general/ltbiandactivetb.htm.

5. Global Tuberculosis Report 2020. World Health Organization. 2020. https://iris.who.int/bitstream/handle/10665/336069 /9789240013131-eng.pdf?sequence=1.

6. Martinez L, Warren JL, Harries AD, et al. Global, Regional, and National Estimates of Tuberculosis Incidence and Case Detection Among Incarcerated Individuals from 2000 to 2019: A Systematic Analysis. *Lancet*. 2023;8(7):E511–E519. https://www.thelancet.com/journals/lanpub/article/PIIS2468 -2667(23)00097-X/fulltext.

7. Placeres AF, de Almeida Soares D, Delpino FM, et al. Epide-miology of TB in Prisoners: A Metanalysis of the Prevalence of Active and Latent TB. *BMC Infectious Diseases*. 2023;23(20). https://bmcinfectdis.biomedcentral.com/articles/10.1186

/s12879-022-07961-8#:~:text=It%20is%20also%20the%20
leading,death%20among%20prisoners%20%5B2%5D;
Centers for Disease Control and Prevention. September 1995.
https://www.cdc.gov/mmwr/preview/mmwrhtml/00042214
.htm.

8.   Signs and Symptoms of Tuberculosis. Centers for Disease
Control and Prevention. March 6, 2024. https://www.cdc.gov
/tb/signs-symptoms/?CDC_AAref_Val=https://www.cdc.gov
/tb/topic/basics/signsandsymptoms.htm.

9.   Walter. Meet Dennis Oya.

10.   Moore R, Schmidt S. Inside the Cell Where a Sick 16-Year-Old
Boy Died in Border Patrol Care. *Propublica*. December 5,
2019. https://www.propublica.org/article/inside-the-cell
-where-a-sick-16-year-old-boy-died-in-border-patrol-care.

11.   Sanchez GV, Bourne CL, Davidson SL, et al. Pneumococcal
Disease Outbreak at a State Prison, Alabama, USA, September 1–October 10, 2018. *EID Journal*. 2021;27(7). https://
wwwnc.cdc.gov/eid/article/27/7/20-3678_t2.

12.   Illness Outbreak Reported at State Prison, 1 Inmate Dead.
Associated Press. September 28, 2018. https://apnews.com
/article/210294ce7bc744bbac6530444707b77d.

13.   Sanchez et al. Pneumococcal Disease Outbreak.

14.   Perfectsublimemasters. Overcrowding in Ventress Prison
During Pandemic, March–July 2020. *Eunoia Review*. October 10, 2020. https://eunoiareview.wordpress.com/2020/10/10
/overcrowding-in-ventress-prison-during-pandemic-march
-july-2020/.

15.   Sanchez et al. Pneumococcal Disease Outbreak.

16.   Alexander M. *The New Jim Crow*. New Press; 2010; Fullilove M. *Root Shock*. New Village Press; 2016.

17.   3 Inmates at York County Jail Test Positive for Tuberculosis.
WSOCTV. October 17, 2023. https://www.wsoctv.com/news
/local/3-inmates-york-county-jail-test-positive-tuberculosis
/TWEVUC25I5EOVPUTC7Y5WMNHLA/.

18. Frieden TR, Fujiwara PI, Washko RM, Hamburg MA. Tuberculosis in New York City—Turning the Tide. *NEJM*. 1995;333(4). https://www.nejm.org/doi/full/10.1056/nejm199 507273330406.

19. Winerip M. On Sunday; Rikers Fights an Epidemic Cell by Cell. *New York Times*. May 24, 1992. https://www.nytimes .com/1992/05/24/nyregion/on-sunday-rikers-fights-an -epidemic-cell-by-cell.html; Sullivan R. Federal Judge Orders Rush on Prison Tuberculosis Unit. *New York Times*. January 25, 1992. https://www.nytimes.com/1992/01/25 /nyregion/federal-judge-orders-rush-on-prison-tuberculosis -unit.html.

20. About Drug Resistant Tuberculosis. Centers for Disease Control and Prevention. December 21, 2023. https://www.cdc .gov/tb/about/drug-resistant.html?CDC_AAref_Val=https:// www.cdc.gov/tb/publications/factsheets/drtb/mdrtb.htm.

21. Sullivan. Federal Judge Orders Rush on Prison Tuberculosis Unit; 2019 Antibiotic Drug Resistance Threats Report. Centers for Disease Control and Prevention. July 16, 2024. https://www.cdc.gov/drugresistance/biggest-threats.html.

22. FAMM—Families for Justice Reform. Accessed April 2024. https://famm.org/; Release Aging People in Prison/RAPP Campaign. Accessed April 2024. https://rappcampaign.com/; Reducing Jail and Prison Populations During the Covid-19 Pandemic. Brennan Center. January 7, 2022. https://www .brennancenter.org/our-work/research-reports/reducing-jail -and-prison-populations-during-covid-19-pandemic; Andress J. Pandemic Inmate Policy Not the Cause of Increased Crime. *Scripps News*. May 17, 2023. https://scrippsnews.com /stories/pandemic-inmate-policy-not-the-cause-of-increased -crime/.

23. Lenthang M. Alabama Inmate Days from Release Dies After Prison Attack Left Him Brain-Dead. *NBC News*. November 14, 2023. https://www.nbcnews.com/news/us-news/alabama -inmate-days-release-dies-prison-attack-left-brain-dead -rcna124866.

24. Rutkoff A. Rikers Fight Club Alleged. *Wall Street Journal.* May 4, 2012. https://www.wsj.com/articles/SB1000142405270 23047528045773845110068841038; Epstein EA. The Real Fight Club at One of America's Toughest Jails. *Daily Mail.* May 6, 2012. https://www.dailymail.co.uk/news/article -2140341/Inside-vicious-fight-club-New-Yorks-Rikers-Island -prison-guards-let-happen.html.

25. Futterman A. 5 Unethical Medical Experiments Brought Out of the Shadows of History. *Discover.* January 11, 2021. https://www.discovermagazine.com/health/5-unethical -medical-experiments-brought-out-of-the-shadows-of -history.

26. California Medical School Apologizes for Unethical Prisoner Experiments. Associated Press. December 23, 2022. https:// www.statnews.com/2022/12/23/ucsf-prisoner-experiments/.

27. Philadelphia Apologizes for Decades of Medical Experiments on Black Inmates That Involved a Component of Agent Orange. Associated Press. October 7, 2022. https://www .nbcnews.com/news/nbcblk/philadelphia-apologizes-decades -medical-experiments-black-inmates-invo-rcna51187.

28. Rapid Increase in Ivermectin Prescriptions and Reports of Severe Illness Associated with Use of Products Containing Ivermectin to Prevent or Treat COVID-19. CDC Health Alert Network. August 26, 2021. https://archive.cdc.gov/#/details ?url=https://emergency.cdc.gov/han/2021/han00449.asp.

29. Crafts L. Ivermectin Experiments in Arkansas Jail Recall Long History of Medical Abuse. *Washington Post.* September 15, 2021. https://www.washingtonpost.com/outlook/2021 /09/15/ivermectin-experiments-an-arkansas-jail-recall-long -history-medical-abuse/.

30. Wood R. Federal Judge Says It's Plausible Karas Experimented on Washington County Jail Detainees, Refuses to Dismiss Lawsuit over Ivermectin. *Arkansas Democrat Gazette.* March 18, 2023. https://www.nwaonline.com/news/2023/mar/18/federal -nwjudge-says-its-plausible-karas/.

31. Darling A. Committee Passes Controversial Resolution
     Honoring Dr. Robert Karas. *KNWA Fox24*. February 7, 2022.
     https://www.nwahomepage.com/news/featured-stories
     /committee-passes-controversial-resolution-honoring-dr
     -robert-karas/; Farar L. Arkansas Medical Board Takes No
     Action Against Jail Doctor Who Treated Inmates with
     Ivermectin for Covid. *Arkansas Democrat Gazette*. June 10,
     2022. https://www.arkansasonline.com/news/2022/jun/10
     /arkansas-medical-board-takes-no-action-against/.

32. "Large" TB Outbreak May Affect 800 People Who Were
     Incarcerated in Washington State. *KOMO News*. December 14,
     2023. https://komonews.com/news/local/washington-tuber
     culosis-prison-outbreak-tb-symptoms-800-incarcerated
     -potentially-exposed-tacoma-pierce-county-health-department
     -cdc-doh-department-of-corrections.

33. A good source of information is the Civil Rights Litigation
     Clearinghouse website at https://clearinghouse.net/. This is a
     resource provided by the University of Michigan Law School
     that allows searching of civil-rights legal cases. I find this site
     extremely helpful because I can see and download expert
     reports and other information about health services that
     come into play as part of litigation. Non-lawyers beware:
     every case has dozens of filings, and finding the content can
     be tricky for those of us who aren't trained, but there are
     often ways to select for the filings that have a .pdf
     attachment.

2. Spider Bite or Staph Infection

1. Throughout this chapter, the details of Mr. Malles's experience
    come from the following document: Court Opinion in Case
    2:06-cv-04024-SD, Filing 86. United States District Court for
    the Eastern District of Pennsylvania. Filed July 27, 2009.
    https://docs.justia.com/cases/federal/district-courts/penn
    sylvania/paedce/2:2006cv04024/210019/86.

2. CDC. Methicillin-Resistant *Staphylococcus aureus* Skin or Soft
    Tissue Infections in a State Prison—Mississippi, 2000. *Morbidity*

and Mortality Weekly Report. October 26, 2001. https://www
.cdc.gov/mmwr/preview/mmwrhtml/mm5042a2.htm.

3.   Photos of MRSA Infections. Centers for Disease Control and
      Prevention. April 15, 2024. https://www.cdc.gov/mrsa
      /communication-resources/photos.html?CDC_AAref_Val
      =https://www.cdc.gov/mrsa/community/photos/index.html.

4.   Lindenmayer J, Schoenfeld S, O'Grady R, Carney JK.
      Methicillin-Resistant Staphylococcus aureus in a High School
      Wrestling Team and the Surrounding Community. *JAMA
      Internal Medicine.* 1998;158(8):895–899. https://jamanetwork
      .com/journals/jamainternalmedicine/fullarticle/191887.

5.   Dixon R. Control of Health-Care-Associated Infections,
      1961–2011. *Morbidity and Mortality Weekly Report.* Octo-
      ber 7, 2011. https://www.cdc.gov/mmwr/preview/mmwrhtml
      /su6004a10.htm.

6.   More Inmates Sue Prison over Infection **MRSA: They Say
      Dirty Conditions in Northampton Jail Led to Spread of
      Disease. *Morning Call.* January 24, 2009. https://www.mcall
      .com/news/mc-xpm-2009-01-24-4294569-story.html.

7.   Summary Judgment in Case 5:12-cv-05323-JD, Document 97.
      United States District Court for the Eastern District of
      Pennsylvania. Filed April 29, 2016. https://www.govinfo.gov
      /content/pkg/USCOURTS-paed-5_12-cv-05323/pdf
      /USCOURTS-paed-5_12-cv-05323-0.pdf.

8.   Dannenberg JE. Two Pennsylvania Prisoners Win $1.2 Million
      For MRSA Skin Infections Contracted County Jail. *Prison
      Legal News.* July 15, 2005. https://www.prisonlegalnews.org
      /news/2005/jul/15/two-pennsylvania-prisoners-win-12
      -million-for-mrsa-skin-infections-contracted-county-jail/.

9.   Ornstein C, Allen JE. Jails See Outbreak of Skin Infections.
      January 31, 2003. *Los Angeles Times.* https://www.latimes
      .com/archives/la-xpm-2003-jan-31-me-staph31-story
      .html#:~:text=%E2%80%9CWe%20spent%20a%20consider
      able%20amount,Sheriff's%20Department's%20chief%20
      medical%20officer.

10. Dannenberg J. Class Action Suit Filed Against L.A. County Jail After 4,000 MRSA Infections. *Prison Legal News.* January 15, 2006. https://www.prisonlegalnews.org/news /2006/jan/15/class-action-suit-filed-against-la-county-jail -after-4000-mrsa-infections/.

11. UCLA Researchers Develop New Model to Predict Spread of "Super-Bug" in L.A. County Jail. *UCLA Health News.* August 17, 2007. https://www.uclahealth.org/news/ucla -researchers-develop-new-model-to-predict-spread-of-super -bug-in-la-county-jail.

12. Managers: Protect Correctional Staff from MRSA. NIOSH Fact Sheet. Centers for Disease Control and Prevention. https://www.cdc.gov/niosh/docs/2013-120/pdfs/2013-120.pdf.

13. Laday J. Cumberland County Pays $125,000 for MRSA Lawsuit. *NJ.com.* July 20, 2011. https://www.nj.com/cumberland/2011/07 /cumberland_county_pays_125000.html.

14. Roos R. Household MRSA Contamination May Fuel Repeat Infections. University of Minnesota Center for Infectious Disease Research and Policy. May 11, 2016. https://www .cidrap.umn.edu/news-perspective/2016/05/household-mrsa -contamination-may-fuel-repeat-infections#:~:text=Patients %20who%20were%20recently%20treated,in%20JAMA%20 Internal%20Medicine%20suggests.

15. Lambert M. IDSA Guidelines on the Treatment of MRSA Infections in Adults and Children. *American Family Physician.* 2011;84(4):455–463. https://www.aafp.org/afp/2011 /0815/p455.html.

16. David MZ, Siegel JD, Henderson J, et al. Hand and Nasal Carriage of Discordant *Staphylococcus aureus* Isolates among Urban Jail Detainees. *J Clin Microbiol.* 2014;52(9):3422– 3425. https://www.ncbi.nlm.nih.gov/pmc/articles/PMC 4313174/.

17. Clinical Overview of MRSA Infection in Healthcare Settings. Centers for Disease Control and Prevention. April 12, 2024. https://www.cdc.gov/mrsa/hcp/clinical-overview/?CDC_AAref _Val=https://www.cdc.gov/mrsa/healthcare/index.html.

18. Brown L, Feuerherd B, Raskin S. Rikers "Emergency" Needs
     Outside Expertise to Replace City Mismanagement, Federal
     Monitor Says. *New York Post*. September 24, 2021. https://
     nypost.com/2021/09/24/rikers-emergency-needs-outside
     -expertise-federal-monitor/; Pinto N. Death on Rikers.
     Intercept. September 21, 2021. https://theintercept.com/2021
     /09/21/death-rikers-island-isa-abdul-karim-crisis-neglect/;
     Sherman R. Rikers Staffing Crisis Limits Access to Medical
     Care. *City*. August 26, 2021. https://www.thecity.nyc/health
     /2021/8/26/22643199/rikers-staffing-crisis-medical-care.

19. Kourtis AP, Hatfield K, Baggs J, et al. Vital Signs: Epidemiol-
     ogy and Recent Trends in Methicillin-Resistant and in
     Methicillin-Susceptible *Staphylococcus aureus* Bloodstream
     Infections—United States. *Morbidity and Mortality Weekly
     Report*. March 8, 2019. https://www.cdc.gov/mmwr/volumes
     /68/wr/mm6809e1.htm; Methicillin-Resistant *Staphylococcus
     aureus*. Fact Sheet. Centers for Disease Control and Preven-
     tion. 2019. https://www.cdc.gov/antimicrobial-resistance
     /media/pdfs/mrsa-508.pdf?CDC_AAref_Val=https://www
     .cdc.gov/drugresistance/pdf/threats-report/mrsa-508.pdf.

20. Malcolm B. The Rise of Methicillin Resistant *Staphylococcus
     aureus* in U.S. Correctional Populations. *J Correct Health
     Care*. 2011;17(3):254–265. https://www.ncbi.nlm.nih.gov/pmc
     /articles/PMC3116074/#:~:text=One%20of%20the%20
     most%20important,for%20MRSA%20infection%20and%20
     colonization.

21. Case 2:02-cv-07377-RB, Filing 23. United States District
     Court for the Eastern District of Pennsylvania. December 23,
     2002. https://clearinghouse.net/doc/34311/.

22. Allen J. Lawsuit: Naples Jail Center Inmate Did Not Receive
     Proper Treatment for Diabetes Before Death. *Naples Daily
     News*. November 12, 2020. https://www.naplesnews.com/story
     /news/crime/2020/11/12/lawsuit-alleges-collier-inmate
     -timothy-kusma-died-after-lack-proper-diabetes-treatment
     /6247046002/.

23. Venters H. Viewpoint: People in New York's Prisons Deserve Better Health Care. *Albany Times Union*. September 21, 2021. https://www.timesunion.com/opinion/article/Viewpoint -People-in-New-York-s-prisons-deserve-16474350.php.

24. Management of Methicillin-Resistant *Staphylococcus aureus* (MRSA) Infections. *Federal Bureau of Prisons Clinical Practice Guidelines*. April 2012. https://www.bop.gov/resources/pdfs /mrsa.pdf.

25. A good source of information is the Civil Rights Litigation Clearinghouse website at https://clearinghouse.net/about.

3. Death and Disability from Outbreaks

1. Florida Jail Prisoner Paralyzed by MRSA Sues Prison Health Services. *Prison Legal News*. April 15, 2010. https://www .prisonlegalnews.org/news/2010/apr/15/florida-jail-prisoner -paralyzed-by-mrsa-sues-prison-health-services/.

2. Florida Jail Prisoner Paralyzed.

3. Fields v. Corizon. Case 11-14594, No. 2:09-cv-00529-JES-DNF. United States Court of Appeals for the Eleventh Circuit. Filed September 6, 2012. https://media.ca11.uscourts.gov/opinions /unpub/files/201114594.pdf.

4. Fields v. Corizon.

5. The company named PHS later became Corizon then YesCare. These changes weren't only cosmetic and involved transitioning through bankruptcy court, which impacted pending settle-ments against the for-profit vendor—which ended up paying out pennies on the dollar for lawsuits over health care. This story was covered in the following reporting: Schwartzapfel B. A Prison Medical Company Faced Lawsuits from Incarcerated People: Then It Went "Bankrupt." *Marshall Project*. Septem-ber 19, 2023. https://www.themarshallproject.org/2023/09/19 /corizon-yescare-private-prison-healthcare-bankruptcy.

6. $1.2 Million Awarded Against PHS After Florida Jail Prisoner Paralyzed. *Prison Legal News*. August 15, 2011. https://www

.prisonlegalnews.org/news/2011/aug/15/12-million-awarded
-against-phs-after-florida-jail-prisoner-paralyzed/.

7. Fields v. Corizon.

8. Fields v. Corizon.

9. Fields v. Corizon.

10. Fields v. Corizon.

11. Glowa-Kollisch S, Graves J, Dickey N, et al. Data-Driven
Human Rights: Using Dual Loyalty Trainings to Promote the
Care of Vulnerable Patients in Jail. *Health and Human Rights
Journal*. 2015;17(1). https://www.hsph.harvard.edu/wp-content
/uploads/sites/2469/2015/06/Venters.pdf.

12. Dual Loyalty in Security Settings: Challenges for Psycholo-
gists. American Psychological Association. Accessed April 1,
2024. https://www.apa.org/education-career/ce/ccw0071.

13. "Solitary confinement" (often called "segregation" by carceral
administrators) refers to being locked in a cell for 22 or more
hours per day. It can be for punitive reasons like being found
guilty in a disciplinary hearing of violating jail or prison rules,
or for administrative reasons like the facility judging a person
to simply be dangerous. Administrative solitary is also used to
punish people without going through an actual disciplinary
hearing and allows for off-the-books punishments.

14. Expert Report of Homer Venters in Case 3:20-cv-00569-MPS,
Document 218-1. United States Court for the District of
Connecticut. Filed September 11, 2020. https://law.yale.edu
/sites/default/files/area/clinic/document/redacted_venters
_report_filed.pdf.

15. Rosenberg R. MCC Officer Made Inmates Perform Sex Acts on
Each Other, Suit Says. *New York Post*. December 4, 2020.
https://nypost.com/2020/12/04/mcc-officer-made-inmates
-perform-sex-acts-on-each-other-suit/; Morales M, Orden E,
Shortell D, Levenson E. 2 Prison Guards Charged with
Conspiracy and Filing False Records on the Night of Jeffrey
Epstein's Death. *CNN*. November 19, 2019. https://www.cnn
.com/2019/11/19/us/jeffrey-epstein-guard-charge/index.html.

16.   As described, in late February 2020, officials received a tip
       that a loaded gun had been smuggled into the facility, possibly
       by staff. As a result, the facility started a two-week process of
       searching every square inch of the building. This required
       transferring many of the detained people to Otisville Correc-
       tional, a facility in Orange County, New York. Eventually, the
       gun was found in the cell of a detained person, which allowed
       the return of people from Otisville. Upon their return, many
       reported that staff conducting the search had broken toilets
       and medical equipment, and had taken clothes and other basic
       property. It was in the wake of this chaos that people started
       to get sick with COVID-19. Reporting on the search for the
       gun can be found here: Dienst J. MCC Returns to Normal
       Operations After Smuggled Gun Triggers Lockdown. *NBC
       New York*. March 11, 2020. https://www.nbcnewyork.com
       /investigations/mcc-returns-to-normal-operations-after
       -smuggled-gun-triggers-8-day-lockdown/2321864/.

17.   Report of Homer Venters and supporting affidavits in
       Fernandez-Rodriguez v. Licon-Vitale. Case 1:20-cv-03315-ER,
       Document 51. United States District Court Southern District of
       New York. Filed May 26, 2020. https://www.fd.org/sites/default
       /files/covid19/bop_jail_policies_and_information/doc_51.pdf.

18.   Expert Report of Homer Venters in Malam v. Adducci. Case
       5:20-cv-10829-JEL-APP, Document 483. United States
       District Court Eastern District of Michigan. Filed January 7,
       2021. https://www.aclumich.org/sites/default/files/field
       _documents/vulnerable_immigrants_freed_from_jail_-
       _malam_v_adducci_-_expert_report.pdf.

19.   Prison Officials Report Death of Inmate at Lompoc Federal
       Correctional Complex. *Santa Maria Times*. December 18, 2020.
       https://santamariatimes.com/news/local/crime-and-courts
       /prison-officials-report-death-of-inmate-at-lompoc-federal
       -correctional-complex/article_bb6c73a0-741a-58a4-ae25
       -141dadc3d82c.html; Inmate Death at FCI Lompoc. Press
       Release. Federal Bureau of Prisons. December 18, 2020.
       https://www.bop.gov/resources/news/pdfs/20201217_press
       _release_lom.pdf.

20. Second Inspection Report of Homer Venters in Torres et al. v. Milusnic et al. Case 2:20-cv-04450-CBM-PVC, Document 239-1. United States District Court, Central District of California. Filed May 12, 2021. https://www.lisa-legalinfo.com /wp-content/uploads/2021/07/VentersReportDkt239 -20cv4450.pdf.

21. Neff J, Kane D. Freed from Prison, Dead from COVID-19, Not Even Counted. *Marshall Project*. July 10, 2020. https://www .themarshallproject.org/2020/07/10/freed-from-prison-dead -from-covid-19-not-even-counted.

22. Blackwell C. Unlocking the Black Box of In-Custody Deaths. *Appeal*. September 6, 2023. https://theappeal.org/death-in -custody-roger-mitchell-jay-aronson/.

23. Jenkins J. Whistleblower: Patients with Mental Illness Suffering in Arizona Prisons. *KJZZ*. June 1, 2018. https://www.kjzz.org /2018-06-01/content-644690-whistleblower-patients-mental -illness-suffering-arizona-prisons.

24. Expert Report of Homer Venters in Harvard v. Inch. Case No. 4:19-cv-00212-W-CAS, Document 311-11. United States District Court Northern District of Florida Tallahassee Division. May 28, 2021. https://storage.courtlistener.com /recap/gov.uscourts.flnd.105133/gov.uscourts.flnd.105133.311 .11.pdf.

25. 2020 Focused Updates to the Asthma Management Guidelines: A Report from the National Asthma Education and Prevention Program Coordinating Committee Expert Panel Working Group. National Heart, Lung, and Blood Institute. December 2020. https://www.nhlbi.nih.gov/resources/2020 -focused-updates-asthma-management-guidelines.

26. The Civil Rights Litigation Clearinghouse website is at https://clearinghouse.net/about.

4. The Farmville Superspreader Event

1. Assessment of COVID-19 Transmission Among Employees and Detained Persons and Infection Prevention & Control Practices at the Farmville Detention Center—Farmville, VA,

June–August 2020: Report September 11, 2020. Centers for Disease Control and Prevention. September 11, 2020. https:// www.wric.com/wp-content/uploads/sites/74/2020/10/CDC -Report-Farmville-Detention-Center-Sept-2020.pdf.

2. Madan MO. Coronavirus Cases Skyrocket at ICE Detention Center in Broward After Transfer from Miami. *Miami Herald.* May 19, 2020. https://www.miamiherald.com/news/local /immigration/article242844451.html; Madan MO. "We May Die and Are Afraid": Federal Judge Makes Public Letters Sent to Him by ICE Detainees. *NNY360.* June 28, 2020. https:// www.nny360.com/news/we-may-die-and-are-afraid-federal -judge-makes-public-letters-sent-to-him-by/article_75522348 -6cd8-5397-a13f-3078dce7d3da.html; Ainsley J, Soboroff J. Nearly Half the Employees at an Arizona ICE Detention Center Have Tested Positive for COVID-19. *NBC News.* July 28, 2020. https://www.nbcnews.com/politics/immigration/nearly -half-employees-arizona-ice-detention-center-have-tested -positive-n1233101.

3. Interim Guidance on Management of Coronavirus Disease 2019 (COVID-19) in Correctional and Detention Facilities. Centers for Disease Control and Prevention. March 27, 2020. https://www.bop.gov/foia/docs//CDCCorrectionalfacilitygui dance3.23.pdf.

4. Declaration of Jeffrey Crawford in Gutierrez v. Hott. Case 1:20-cv-00712-LMB-IDD, Document 13-1. United States District Court Eastern District of Virginia. Filed July 9, 2020. https://www.wric.com/wp-content/uploads/sites/74/2020/07 /0013-001.-07-09-2020-Crawford-Declaration-highlighted.pdf.

5. Declaration of Jeffrey Crawford.

6. Expert Report of Homer Venters in Case 1:20-cv-00821-LMB -JFA, Document 79-1. United States District Court Eastern District of Virginia. Filed September 4, 2020. https://nipnlg .org/work/resources/santos-garcia-et-al-v-wolf-et-al-inspection -report.

7. Canadian Man in ICE Custody Passes Away in Virginia. Press Release. US Immigration and Customs Enforcement. August 7,

2020. https://www.ice.gov/news/releases/canadian-man-ice
-custody-passes-away-virginia.

8.   Canadian Man in ICE Custody Passes Away in Virginia.

9.   Moreno S. "It's a Story That Shouldn't Have Happened":
     72-Year-Old Man in Farmville ICE Facility Dies After Testing
     Positive for COVID-19. *Richmond Times-Dispatch*. August 7,
     2020. https://richmond.com/news/virginia/its-a-story-that
     -shouldnt-have-happened-72-year-old-man-in-farmville-ice
     -facility/article_643fec10-cb95-5fed-af89-3b248338a162.
     html.

10. Interim Guidance on Management of Coronavirus Disease
     2019 (COVID-19) in Correctional and Detention Facilities.

11. Canadian Man in ICE Custody Passes Away in Virginia.

12. Expert Report of Homer Venters.

13. Expert Report of Homer Venters. This question, whether the
     sick-call requests result in timely care, is a common metric in
     detention settings, and my experience monitoring this is that
     100% compliance is rarely if ever achieved. Even in the best of
     times, there are some delays in seeing people who request care,
     given the security setting. During COVID-19, this often-
     deficient system was under even more pressure because of
     restrictions on people's movement to see nurses and doctors,
     and because of short staffing.

14. Expert Report of William Reese in Case 1:20-cv-00821-LMB
     -JFA, Document 81. United States District Court Eastern
     District of Virginia Alexandria Division. Filed September 4,
     2020. https://www.courtlistener.com/docket/17372814/santos
     -garcia-v-wolf/.

15. Assessment of COVID-19 Transmission Among Employees
     and Detained Persons.

16. Expert Report of Homer Venters.

17. Assessment of COVID-19 Transmission Among Employees
     and Detained Persons.

18. Expert Report of Homer Venters.

19. Farmville Town Council Meeting. *Facebook*. August 12, 2020. https://www.facebook.com/farmillevagov/videos/town-council-meeting-august-122020/2777893755820049/.

20. Expert Report of Homer Venters.

21. Assessment of COVID-19 Transmission Among Employees and Detained Persons.

22. Lemieux JE, Siddle KJ, Shaw BM, et al. Phylogenetic Analysis of SARS-CoV-2 in Boston Highlights the Impact of Super-spreading Events. *Science*. 2020;371(6529). https://science.sciencemag.org/content/early/2020/12/09/science.abe3261.full.

23. Olivo A, Miroff N. ICE Flew Detainees to Virginia So Planes Could Transport Agents to DC Protests. A Huge Coronavirus Outbreak Followed. *Washington Post*. September 11, 2020. https://www.washingtonpost.com/coronavirus/ice-air-farmville-protests-covid/2020/09/11/f70ebe1e-e861-11ea-bc79-834454439a44_story.html.

24. Olivo, Miroff. ICE Flew Detainees to Virginia.

25. Winter J. Exclusive: Leaked Document Reveals Details of Federal Law Enforcement Patrolling Washington amid Protests. *Yahoo News*. June 5, 2020. https://news.yahoo.com/exclusive-leaked-document-reveals-details-of-federal-law-enforcement-patrolling-washington-amid-protests-154138680.html?guccounter=1.

26. Olivo, Miroff. ICE Flew Detainees to Virginia.

27. Olivo, Miroff. ICE Flew Detainees to Virginia.

28. Farmville Town Council Meeting.

29. The Dark Money Trail Behind Private Detention: Immigration Centers of America—Farmville. National Immigrant Justice Center. October 2019. https://immigrantjustice.org/sites/default/files/content-type/research-item/documents/2019-10/NIJC-policy-brief_ICA-Farmville_Oct2019.pdf.

30. Immigration and Customs Enforcement Did Not Follow Federal Procurement Guidelines When Contracting for Detention Services. US Department of Homeland Security

Office of Inspector General. Report OIG-18-53. February 21, 2018. https://www.oig.dhs.gov/sites/default/files/assets/2018 -02/OIG-18-53-Feb18.pdf.

31. Expert Report of Homer Venters.

32. Capstone Review of the Federal Bureau of Prisons' Response to the Coronavirus Disease 2019 Pandemic. Federal Bureau of Prisons Office of Inspector General. Report 23-054. March 2023. https://oig.justice.gov/sites/default/files/reports /23-054.pdf.

33. Many Factors Hinder ICE's Ability to Maintain Adequate Medical Staffing at Detention Facilities. US Department of Homeland Security Office of Inspector General. Report 22-03. October 29, 2021. https://www.oig.dhs.gov/sites/default/files /assets/2021-11/OIG-22-03-Oct21.pdf.

34. Refer to the Civil Rights Litigation Clearinghouse website at https://clearinghouse.net/about.

5. Heat

1. Foxhall E. Family Sues TDCJ over Heat-Related Death. *Texas Tribune*. June 26, 2012. https://www.texastribune.org/2012 /06/26/tdcj-files-wrongful-death-lawsuit/.

2. The details about Mr. McCollum's experience come from the following document: Civil Complaint in Case 4:14-cv-3253. United States District Court Southern District of Texas. Filed February 3, 2017. https://casetext.com/case/mccollum-v -livingston-1.

3. Memorandum and Order. Civil Complaint in Case 4:14-cv- 3253, Document 342. United States District Court Southern District of Texas. Filed February 3, 2017. https://casetext.com /case/mccollum-v-livingston-1.

4. Banks G. Judge's Order Hits State Hard over Heat-Related Inmate Deaths. *Houston Chronicle*. February 14, 2017. https://www.houstonchronicle.com/news/houston-texas /houston/article/Judge-s-order-hits-state-hard-over-heat -related-10932997.php.

5. Principles of Epidemiology, Glossary. Centers for Disease Control. Archived Page. https://archive.cdc.gov/www_cdc_gov /csels/dsepd/ss1978/glossary.html#:~:text=outbreak%20 the%20occurrence%20of%20more,persons%20during%20 a%20specific%20period.

6. McCullough J. "It's a Living Hell": Scorching Heat in Texas Prisons Revives Air-Conditioning Debate. *Texas Tribune.* August 24, 2022. https://www.texastribune.org/2022/08/24 /texas-prisons-air-conditioning/; McCullough J. Despite Budget Surplus, Texas Legislature Makes Little Money Available for Prison Air Conditioning. *Texas Tribune.* May 26, 2023. https://www.texastribune.org/2023/05/26/texas -prisons-air-conditioning/.

7. McCullough J. Judge Approves Settlement Mandating Air Conditioning at Hot Texas Prison. *Texas Tribune.* May 8, 2018. https://www.texastribune.org/2018/05/08/settlement-air -condition-hot-texas-prison-gets-final-judicial-approval/; Complaint in Case 4:14-cv-01698, Document 1449. United States District Court Southern District of Texas. Filed August 9, 2019. https://storage.courtlistener.com/recap/gov .uscourts.txsd.1184918/gov.uscourts.txsd.1184918.1449.0_1.pdf.

8. Blakinger K. Federal Judge Dings Texas Prison System for Violating Terms of Settlement in Lawsuit over Sweltering Prisons. *Houston Chronicle.* August 10, 2012. https://www .houstonchronicle.com/news/houston-texas/houston/article /Federal-judge-dings-Texas-prison-system-for-14295678.php.

9. McCullough J. "It's a Living Hell": Scorching Heat; McCullough J. Despite Budget Surplus.

10. TDCJ Air Conditioning Projects. Texas Department of Criminal Justice. Accessed June 15, 2024. https://www.tdcj .texas.gov/ac/index.html.

11. Indicator: Heat-Related Mortality. National Environmental Public Health Tracking Network. Centers for Disease Control and Prevention. Accessed June 15, 2024. https://ephtracking .cdc.gov/indicatorPages?selectedContentAreaAbbreviation =35&selectedIndicatorId=67; Centers for Disease Control and

Prevention. Heat-Related Deaths—United States, 2004–2018. *Morbidity and Mortality Weekly Report*. June 19, 2020. https://www.cdc.gov/mmwr/volumes/69/wr/mm6924a1.htm.

12. See search results for "prison heat" on the *Texas Tribune* website. Accessed December 30, 2023. https://www .texastribune.org/search/?q=prison+heat#gsc.tab=0&gsc.q =prison%20heat&gsc.page=1.

13. Civil Complaint in Case 4:14-cv-3253.

14. Civil Complaint in Case 4:14-cv-3253.

15. McCullough J. A State Report Says a Texas Inmate Died from Heat Last Year. Prison Officials Contest That Finding. *Texas Tribune*. February 19, 2019. https://www.texastribune.org /2019/02/19/texas-prison-heat-death/.

16. Civil Complaint in Case 4:14-cv-3253.

17. Vassalo S. Report on the Risks of Heat-Related Illness and Access to Medical Care for Death Row Inmates Confined to Unit 32, Mississippi State Penitentiary, Parchman, Mississippi. For American Civil Liberties Union's National Prison Project. September 2002. https://www.aclu.org/sites/default /files/pdfs/prison/vassallo_report.pdf.

18. Settlement Agreement in Case 75 Civ. 3073 (HB) (SDNY) United States District Court, Southern District New York. Filed October 6, 2008. https://casetext.com/case/benjamin-v-horn.

19. Skarha J, Dominick A, Spangler K, et al. Provision of Air Conditioning and Heat-Related Mortality in Texas Prisons. *JAMA Network Open*. 2022;5(11) e2239849. https:// jamanetwork.com/journals/jamanetworkopen/fullarticle /2798097.

20. Texas Says No Inmates Have Died Due to Stifling Heat in Its Prisons Since 2012. Some Data May Suggest Otherwise. *CBS News*. July 19, 2023. https://www.cbsnews.com/news/texas -prisons-heat-deaths-disputed-claims-inmate-families -worry/.

21. Skarha et al. Provision of Air Conditioning.

22. Flahive P. Texas Claims Spike in Prison Deaths Isn't Heat-Related. Study Says That Can't Be True. *Texas Public Radio.* August 9, 2023. https://www.tpr.org/criminal-justice/2023 -08-09/a-spike-in-deaths-hits-texas-prisons-as-study -challenges-states-claim-of-no-heat-related-deaths; Weill-Greenberg E, Wing N. Extreme Heat Is Killing People in Prison. What's Being Done About It? *Appeal.* August 29, 2023. https://theappeal.org/heat-prison-deaths-air -conditioning/; Baker A. "Air Conditioning Is a Human Right." Heat-Related Prison Deaths Are Rising Due to Climate Change. *Time.* May 23, 2023. https://time.com /6281702/prisons-heat-deaths-climate-change-air -conditioning/.

23. Hernandez A. Stifling Prison Heat Used to Be Just a Southern Problem. Not Anymore. *Washington State Standard.* August 14, 2023. https://washingtonstatestandard.com/2023/08 /14/stifling-prison-heat-used-to-be-just-a-southern-problem -not-anymore/.

24. O'Dea C. Heat Waves Spur NJ Prison Watchdog, Who Says Thousands of Cells "Dangerously Hot." *NJ Spotlight News.* September 6, 2022. https://www.njspotlightnews.org/2022 /09/new-jersey-corrections-ombudsman-urges-state -improve-living-conditions-heat-waves-air-conditioning/; Shuster T, King K. Special Report: Summer Heat in New Jersey Prisons. New Jersey Office of the Corrections Ombudsperson. September 6, 2022. https://www.nj.gov/corrections ombudsperson/documents/Jail%20Inspection%20Reports /DOC%20Ombudsperson%20Special%20Report-%20Heat .pdf.

25. Sax S. Like Sitting in a Sauna: Heat Waves Cause Misery in WA Prisons. *PBS.* June 9, 2022. https://www.cascadepbs.org /equity/2022/06/sitting-sauna-heat-waves-cause-misery-wa -prisons; Maynes J. Walla Walla Breaks All-Time Heat Record. *Union-Bulletin.* June 30, 2021. https://www.union -bulletin.com/news/walla-walla-breaks-all-time-heat-record /article_64c81560-d9af-11eb-9b16-cbf08e192237.html.

26. Captive Labor: Exploitation of Incarcerated Workers. American Civil Liberties Union. June 15, 2022. https://www.aclu.org/news/human-rights/captive-labor-exploitation-of-incarcerated-workers.

27. Fassler E. For Incarcerated Workers, Summer Heat Can Be a Death Sentence. *In These Times*. August 28, 2019. https://inthesetimes.com/article/incarcerated-workers-prison-dangerous-heat-work-conditions; Hauptman M. The Health and Safety of Incarcerated Workers: OSHA's Applicability in the Prison Context. *ABA Journal of Labor & Employment Law*. 2023;37(1). https://www.americanbar.org/content/dam/aba/publications/aba_journal_of_labor_employment_law/v37/no-1/jlel-37-1-5.pdf.

28. Heat: Personal Risk Factors. Occupational Safety and Health Administration. Accessed June 15, 2024. https://www.osha.gov/heat-exposure/personal-risk-factors and https://www.osha.gov/sites/default/files/publications/OSHA3975.pdf.

29. Rosenfeld J. The Origin of Prisoner's Rights: Estelle v. Gamble 429 U.S. 97; 75-929 (1976). *National Law Review*. September 16, 2016. https://www.natlawreview.com/article/origin-prisoner-s-rights-estelle-v-gamble-429-us-97-75-929-1976.

30. Lozano J. Judge Threatens to Bring the Heat to Texas Prison Officials. Associated Press. September 6, 2019. https://apnews.com/c36647e388234f3db8ef40036ceb1059.

31. Documents: Officials Knew About Rikers Heat Problem Before Inmate's Death. *CBS News New York*. May 6, 2014. https://www.cbsnews.com/newyork/news/documents-officials-knew-about-rikers-heat-problem-before-inmates-death/.

32. Guard Arrested in Death of NYC Inmate in Hot Cell. *CBS News New York*. December 9, 2014. https://www.cbsnews.com/news/guard-arrested-in-death-of-nyc-inmate-in-hot-cell/.

33. Ex-Marine's Heat Death in NYC Jail Ruled Accidental. *CBS News*. September 12, 2014. https://www.cbsnews.com/news/ex-marines-nyc-jail-death-ruled-accidental/.

34. Associated Press. Pennsylvania Prison Salmonella Outbreak Sickened 300. *Syracuse.com*. July 15, 2011. https://www .syracuse.com/news/2011/07/pennsylvani_prison_salmonella .html.

35. Gicquelais RE, Morris JF, Matthews HS, et al. Multiple-Serotype Salmonella Outbreaks in Two State Prisons— Arkansas, August 2012. *Morbidity and Mortality Weekly Report*. February 28, 2014. https://www.cdc.gov/mmwr /preview/mmwrhtml/mm6308a2.htm?s_cid=mm6308a2_w.

36. Gicquelais et al. Multiple-Serotype Salmonella Outbreaks.

37. Marlow MA, Luna-Gierke RE, Griffin PM, Vieira AR. Food-borne Disease Outbreaks in Correctional Institutions—United States, 1998–2014. *Am J Public Health*. 2017;107(7);1150–1156. https://www.ncbi.nlm.nih.gov/pmc/articles/PMC5463225/.

38. Lewis T. Bird Flu Detected in Humans in the US: What We Know So Far. *Scientific American*. April 2, 2024. https://www .scientificamerican.com/article/bird-flu-detected-in-a-person -in-texas-what-we-know-so-far.

39. In 2024, the Associated Press did an incredible investigation of prison work that included following groups of workers from prisons to farms and other work settings, revealing a supply chain of labor and products that stretches from state prisons into Target, Walmart, Kroger, and Kellogg's Frosted Flakes. Reporting for this story can be found at McDowell R, Mason M. Prisoners in the US Are Part of a Hidden Workforce Linked to Hundreds of Popular Food Brands. Associated Press. January 29, 2024. https://apnews.com/article/prison-to-plate -inmate-labor-investigation-c6f0eb4747963283316e494e adf08c4e.

40. Nigra AE, Navas-Acien A. Arsenic in US Correctional Facility Drinking Water, 2006–2011. *Environ Res*. 2020;188:109768. https://www.ncbi.nlm.nih.gov/pmc/articles/PMC7483613/; Townsend-Lerdo E, Claudy I. 5 Stories About Unhealthy Water Inside Prisons. *Prison Journalism Project*. October 11, 2023. https://prisonjournalismproject.org/2023/10/11/five -stories-unsafe-drinking-water-prisons/; Haney A. Elevated

Levels of Arsenic Found at Federal Penitentiary in Atlanta. *11 Alive.* February 7, 2019. https://www.11alive.com/article/news /elevated-levels-of-arsenic-found-at-federal-penitentiary-in -atlanta/85-ecf4c149-a800-4295-a1b1-6ea8d56bf3af.

41. Investigation Reveals Environmental Dangers in America's Toxic Prisons. Equal Justice Initiative. June 16, 2017. https:// eji.org/news/investigation-reveals-environmental-dangers-in -toxic-prisons/; Manke K. Study Finds Potentially Dangerous Levels of Arsenic in Prison Drinking Water. *Berkeley News.* September 21, 2022. https://news.berkeley.edu/2022/09/21 /study-finds-potentially-dangerous-levels-of-arsenic-in-prison -drinking-water.

42. Centers for Disease Control and Prevention. Notes from the Field: Botulism from Drinking Prison-Made Illicit Alcohol— Arizona, 2012. *Morbidity and Mortality Weekly Report.* 2013;62(05):88.https://www.cdc.gov/mmwr/preview /mmwrhtml/mm6205a3.htm.

43. Marlow M, Edwards L, McCrickard L, et al. Mild Botulism from Illicitly Brewed Alcohol in a Large Prison Outbreak in Mississippi. *Frontiers in Public Health.* 2021;9(21). https://www.frontiersin.org/articles/10.3389/fpubh.2021 .716615/full.

44. Uranga F. Limited Regulations Make Texas Workers Responsible for Preventing On-the-Job Heat Injuries. *Texas Tribune.* July 12, 2023. https://www.texastribune.org/2023/07/12 /workers-texas-heat-wave/.

45. Centers for Disease Control and Prevention. Heat-Related Mortality—Chicago, July 1995. *Morbidity Mortality Weekly Report.* 1995;44(31):577–579. https://www.cdc.gov/mmwr /preview/mmwrhtml/00038443.htm.

46. Overdose Deaths and Jail Incarceration. National Trends and Racial Disparities. Vera. Accessed June 15, 2024. https://www .vera.org/publications/overdose-deaths-and-jail-incarceration /national-trends-and-racial-disparities.

47. The Civil Rights Litigation Clearinghouse website can be found at https://clearinghouse.net/about.

48. Arshad M. Lawsuit Says Prison Labor System in Alabama Amounts to "Modern-Day Form of Slavery." *USA Today.* December 14, 2023. https://www.usatoday.com/story/news /nation/2023/12/14/alabama-prison-labor-modern-slavery /71898583007/.

6. The Incredible Itch

1. Civil Complaint in Case 3:17-cv-00949, Document 1. United States District Court Middle District Tennessee at Nashville. Filed June 17, 2017. https://clearinghouse-umich-production .s3.amazonaws.com/media/doc/100319.pdf.

2. About Scabies. Centers for Disease Control and Prevention. February 23, 2024. https://www.cdc.gov/scabies/about/?CDC _AAref_Val; Scabies. World Health Organization. May 31, 2023. https://www.who.int/news-room/fact-sheets/detail /scabies#:~:text=Scabies%20can%20lead%20to%20 skin,in%20low%2Dincome%20tropical%20areas.

3. Da Silva LJ. The Etymology of *Infection* and *Infestation*. *Pediatric Infect Dis J.* 1997;16(12):1188. https://journals.lww .com/pidj/fulltext/1997/12000/the_etymology_of_infection _and_infestation.23.aspx#:~:text=Infest%20conveys%20 the%20idea%20of,included%2C%20but%20attack%20 with%20penetration.

4. Pierrotti A. Former Model Eaten Alive by Scabies in Georgia Nursing Home. *USA Today.* April 28, 2018. https://www .usatoday.com/story/money/nation-now/2018/04/28/former -model-eaten-alive-scabies-georgia-nursing-home/561394002/.

5. Pierotti. Former Model Eaten Alive.

6. Brown M. CoreCivic Settles Lawsuit over Nashville Jail Scabies Outbreak. *Nashville Tennessean.* December 8, 2021. https:// www.tennessean.com/story/news/2021/12/08/corecivic-settles -lawsuit-over-nashville-jail-scabies-outbreak/8827935002/.

7. Barchenger S. Emails: Scabies at Nashville Jail Treated in January; Doctors Blame Mold. https://www.tennessean.com /story/news/2017/06/14/emails-scabies-nashville-jail-treated -january-doctors-blame-mold/391866001/.

8. Civil Complaint in Case 3:17-cv-00949, Document 1.

9. Civil Complaint in Case 3:17-cv-00949, Document 36. United States District Court Middle District Tennessee at Nashville. Filed June 27, 2018. https://law.justia.com/cases/federal /district-courts/tennessee/tnmdce/3:2017cv00949/71147/36/.

10. Egan P. How Flint MD Solved Rash Mystery That Stumped Women's Prison Officials. *Detroit Free Press.* January 18, 2019. https://www.freep.com/story/news/local/michigan/2019/01/18 /flint-doctor-walter-barkey-womens-prison-scabies/25953 24002/.

11. Egan. How Flint MD Solved Rash Mystery.

12. Shamus KJ. Flint Dermatologists Volunteer to Help Diagnose Rashes. *Detroit Free Press.* March 6, 2016. https://www.freep .com/story/news/2016/03/06/flint-dermatologists-volunteer -help-diagnose-rashes/81336528/.

13. Scabies Skin Scraping Procedure. Los Angeles Department of Public Health. Accessed April 2024. http://publichealth .lacounty.gov/acd/docs/Scabies/ScabiesAppendixC.pdf.

14. Egan. How Flint MD Solved Rash Mystery.

15. Civil Complaint in Case 3:17-cv-00949, Document 36.

16. Civil Complaint in Case 3:17-cv-00949, Document 36.

17. Civil Complaint in Case 3:17-cv-00949, Document 36.

18. Know Your Rights: The Prison Litigation Reform Act (PLRA). American Civil Liberties Union. Accessed April 2024. https://www.aclu.org/sites/default/files/images/asset_upload _file79_25805.pdf.

19. In many detention settings, a person fills out a sick-call form on paper or electronically. The exact information they send to the facility should end up in their medical records but often doesn't, so that the first record of their medical problem occurs when they are seen, which could be much later and may omit the symptoms and other exact details they sent in.

20. Civil Case 2:19-cv-10707-VAR-PTM. ECF-69. United States District Court for the Eastern District of Michigan Southern

Division. Filed February 20, 2020. https://irp.cdn-website
.com/b5bb3176/files/uploaded/Amended%20Scabies.pdf;
Schwartzapfel B. A Prison Medical Company Faced Lawsuits
from Incarcerated People. Then It Went "Bankrupt." *USA
Today*. September 19, 2023. https://www.usatoday.com/story
/news/nation/2023/09/19/corizon-yescare-private-prison
-healthcare-bankruptcy/70892593007/.

21. Civil Case 2:19-cv-10707-VAR-PTM. ECF-109. United States
District Court for the Eastern District of Michigan Southern
Division. Filed August 24, 2020. https://law.justia.com/cases
/federal/district-courts/michigan/miedce/2:2019cv10707
/336818/109/.

22. A Google search for the words "scabies" and "prison" yielded
93 results under the "News" tab on August 27, 2024. When
"prison" was changed to "jail," there were 55 results.

23. Civil Complaint in Case 3:17-cv-00949, Document 36.

24. Another thing that struck me about the court screening room
was that it was down a short flight of stairs from the hallway
where people would wait, standing in a row while cuffed. Anyone
with a disability or injury or who was too frail to go down those
stairs would just stay at the top while the EMTs yelled their
screening questions to them. Many of the clinic spaces I've seen
across prisons and jails also have this problem—they are
inaccessible for people with injuries or disabilities. The first
health screening that happens when a person gets into a prison
or jail, sometimes called the "receiving screening," occurs while a
person is standing somewhere in the facility intake, in full
earshot of security staff. Without the ability to speak confidentially, patients are less likely to report their health issues,
especially mental-health and substance-use problems.

25. Speaking with the person identified as an infection-control
nurse or officer is important to determine their scope and time
commitment in this area. In my experience, an infection-
control nurse, a disability or Americans with Disabilities Act
coordinator, and a sexual assault or Prison Rape Elimination
Act coordinator are three roles that almost always exist on

paper but are often underfunded or unfilled. A facility may be able to give the name of a person with the title, but it's important to dig in to what percentage of their work time is allocated to this role.

26.   The Civil Rights Litigation Clearinghouse website can be found at https://clearinghouse.net/about.

7. Independent Inspections During Outbreaks

1.   Expert Report of Homer Venters in Case 2:20-cv-02359 SHL. United States District Court for the Western District of Tennessee. Filed July 9, 2020. https://clearinghouse.net/case /17614/.

2.   Sainz A. 6 of 9 Deputies Plead Not Guilty to Charges in Death of Gershun Freeman in Memphis Jail. *ABC News*. October 27, 2023. https://www.localmemphis.com/article/news/crime /shelby-county-corrections-deputies-arraigned-charges -death-gershun-freeman/522-661214f9-1b1b-43ec-8c07 -5bdfada52130; Finton L. Footage from Jail Shows Officers Kneeling on Gershun Freeman's Back for Almost 6 Minutes. *Commercial Appeal*. March 2, 2023. https://www.commercia lappeal.com/story/news/2023/03/02/video-released-of-shelby -county-jail-officers-beating-inmate/69964005007/.

3.   Expert Report of Homer Venters.

4.   Expert Report of Homer Venters.

5.   Groups File Lawsuit Against Shelby County Jail Seeking Release of Those Most at Risk of COVID. Press Release. ACLU of Tennessee. May 20, 2020. https://www.aclu.org/press-releases /groups-file-lawsuit-against-shelby-county-jail-seeking-release -those-most-risk-covid.

6.   Expert Report of Michael Brady in Case 2:20-cv-02359 SHL. United States District Court for the Western District of Tennessee. Filed June 29, 2020. https://clearinghouse.net/case/17614/.

7.   Advocates Reach Agreement with Shelby County Sheriff to Fix Dangerous Pandemic Jail Conditions. Press Release. ACLU of Tennessee. April 9, 2021. https://www.aclu.org/press-releases

/advocates-reach-agreement-shelby-county-sheriff-fix
-dangerous-pandemic-jail.

8. Expert Report of Owen Murray in Case 7:20-cv-00062-
    CDL-MSH. United States District Court for the Middle
    District of Georgia Valdosta Division, Document 75–1. Filed
    May 27, 2020.

9. Expert Report of Owen Murray.

10. Project South, Georgia Detention Watch, Georgia Latino
    Alliance for Human Rights, South Georgia Immigrant Support
    Network to Cuffari JV, Quinn C, Giles TP, Paulk D. Re: Lack of
    Medical Care, Unsafe Work Practices, and Absence of Adequate
    Protection Against COVID-19 for Detained Immigrants and
    Employees Alike at the Irwin County Detention Center. Septem-
    ber 14, 2020. https://projectsouth.org/wp-content/uploads
    /2020/09/OIG-ICDC-Complaint-1.pdf.

11. Boone C, Mitchell T. ICE Cuts Ties to SW Georgia Immigrant
    Detention Facility. *Atlanta Journal-Constitution*. May 20,
    2021. https://www.ajc.com/news/crime/ice-cuts-ties-to-sw
    -georgia-immigrant-detention-facility/725XZELXJFBV7GSK
    DEC6YVAVII/; Shoichet CE. Four Women Are Accusing a
    Nurse at an ICE Detention Center of Sexual Assault. *CNN*.
    July 15, 2022. https://www.cnn.com/2022/07/14/us/ice
    -stewart-detention-center-nurse-assault-allegations/index
    .html.

12. The Mental Health Care System in Alabama's Prisons.
    Southern Poverty Law Center. Accessed April 2024. https://
    www.splcenter.org/sites/default/files/factsheet_cjr_the
    _mental_health_care_system_in_alabama_s_prisons.pdf.

13. The Mental Health Care System.

14. State's Response to Inspections in Case 2:14-cv-00601-MHT-
    JTA, Document 2993. United States District Court for the
    Middle District of Alabama Northern Division. Filed Septem-
    ber 28, 2020. https://clearinghouse.net/case/15211/.

15. Court Opinion in Case 2:14-cv-00601-MHT-JTA, Document
    3046. United States District Court for the Middle District of

Alabama Northern Division. Filed October 29, 2020. https://www.alreporter.com/wp-content/uploads/2020/10/plaintiffs.pdf.

16. Justice Department Alleges Conditions at Massachusetts Department of Correction Violate the Constitution. Press Release. US Attorney's Office, District of Massachusetts. November 17, 2020. https://www.justice.gov/usao-ma/pr/justice-department-alleges-conditions-massachusetts-department-correction-violate.

17. Department of Justice Takes Legal Action to Address Pattern and Practice of Excessive Force and Violence at Rikers Island Jails That Violates the Constitutional Rights of Young Male Inmates. Press Release. US Attorney's Office, Southern District of New York. December 18, 2014. https://www.justice.gov/usao-sdny/pr/department-justice-takes-legal-action-address-pattern-and-practice-excessive-force-and.

18. Nunez Monitor Reports. New York City Department of Correction. Accessed June 15, 2024. https://www.nyc.gov/site/doc/media/nunez-reports.page; Kaye J. Rikers Monitor Says Relationship with DOC Has "Eroded." *Queens Daily Eagle*. December 4, 2023. https://queenseagle.com/all/2023/12/4/rikers-monitor-says-relationship-with-doc-has-eroded.

19. Stroud H. The Way Forward for Rikers Island: Receivership. Brennan Center for Justice. January 4, 2022. https://www.brennancenter.org/our-work/analysis-opinion/way-forward-rikers-island-receivership.

20. FAQ About Pattern or Practice Investigations. US Department of Justice Civil Rights Division. https://www.justice.gov/d9/2023-10/pattern_or_practice_investigation_faqs_english.pdf.

21. Emerson J. Why 20 Hospitals Have Been at Risk of Losing CMS Funding. *Becker's Hospital Review*. December 19, 2023. https://www.beckershospitalreview.com/hospital-finance/why-9-hospitals-have-been-at-risk-of-losing-cms-funding.html.

22. By comparison, state governments have clear regulations about how health systems must maintain accreditation based

on public standards and measurements. For example, see this website with criteria for New York: https://www.health.ny.gov/facilities/hospital/accreditation/; and this website for Texas: https://www.hhs.texas.gov/providers/health-care-facilities-regulation/hospitals-general-hospitals.

23. Preventing Torture: The Role of National Preventive Mechanisms. United Nations, Human Rights, Office of the High Commissioner. 2018. https://www.ohchr.org/Documents/HRBodies/OPCAT/NPM/NPM_Guide.pdf.

24. Subcommittee on Prevention of Torture. United Nations, Human Rights, Office of the High Commissioner. Accessed June 15, 2024. https://www.ohchr.org/en/hrbodies/opcat/pages/opcatindex.aspx.

25. Van den Bergh B, Michaelsen L, Brasholt M, Modvig J. Monitoring Health in Places of Detention. Dignity—Danish Institute Against Torture. 2021. https://dignity.dk/wp-content/uploads/DIGNITY-Health-Monitoring-Manual_WEB-ENG-V.1.1.pdf.

26. Suicides in San Diego County Jail: A System Failing People with Mental Illness. Disability Rights California. April 25, 2018. https://www.disabilityrightsca.org/public-reports/san-diego-jail-suicides-report; Inmate Rights Under the Americans with Disabilities Act: A Brief Overview. Disability Rights Pennsylvania. 2018. https://www.disabilityrightspa.org/wp-content/uploads/2018/04/ADA-2E-Inmste-Rights-ADA.pdf.

27. What We Do. Disability Rights New York. Accessed June 15, 2024. https://www.drny.org/page/what-we-do-6.html#:~:text=DRNY%20is%20the%20federally%20and,services%20to%20individuals%20with%20disabilities.

28. Class Settlement Agreement Notice in Case 3:30-CV-534 (JBA). United States District Court District of Connecticut. Filed June 17, 2020. https://portal.ct.gov/-/media/doc/pdf/coronavirus-3-20/notice-to-the-class-re-settlement-of-covid19-related-lawsuit-062320.pdf.

29. McPherson v. Lamont Settlement Documents. ACLU Connecticut. Accessed June 15, 2024. https://www.acluct.org/en/mcpherson-v-lamont-settlement-documents.

30. Dayton K. Panel Will Oversee Efforts by Prisons and Jails to Manage Pandemic Threat. *Honolulu Civil Beat.* September 3, 2021. https://www.civilbeat.org/2021/09/panel-will-oversee -efforts-by-prisons-and-jails-to-manage-pandemic-threat/.

31. Learn about the Civil Rights Litigation Clearinghouse at https://clearinghouse.net/about.

8. Saving Lives During Outbreaks

1. Phillips K. Woman Who Was Arrested After Missing Officials' Phone Call While in Computer Class Is Headed Home. *USA Today.* July 6, 2021. https://www.usatoday.com/story/news /politics/2021/07/06/gwen-levi-headed-home-after-judge -approves-compassionate-release/7877359002/.

2. Reinhart E, Chen DL. Incarceration and Its Disseminations: COVID-19 Pandemic Lessons from Chicago's Cook County Jail. *Health Affairs.* 2020;39(8). https://www.healthaffairs.org /doi/10.1377/hlthaff.2020.00652.

3. Reinhart E, Chen DL. Carceral-Community Epidemiology, Structural Racism, and COVID-19 Disparities. *PNAS.* 2021;118(21). https://www.pnas.org/doi/10.1073/pnas.2026 577118.

4. Walsh C. Study Suggests New Lessons on COVID-19 and Mass Incarceration. *Harvard Gazette.* June 9, 2021. https://news .harvard.edu/gazette/story/2021/06/study-sheds-new-light-on -covid-19-and-mass-incarceration/.

5. Clostridium Difficile Campaign. Illinois Department of Public Health. Accessed June 15, 2024. https://dph.illinois.gov/topics -services/prevention-wellness/patient-safety-quality/cdiff -campaign.html; *Clostridium difficile* Infection in the Chicago Area: Classification, Epidemiology, and Health Care Facility Rates, February 2009. *CDInfo.* August 2009. https://www .chicagohan.org/documents/14171/23731/(082009)+Clostridium +difficile+infection+in+the+Chicago+area.pdf/80dffa70-bf2b -4fb3-8b65-c16261f89574.

6. See the State Prison Overcrowding page and map from 2019 at the University of Nebraska Omaha's website: https://www

.unomaha.edu/college-of-public-affairs-and-community-service
/governing/stories/state-prison-overcrowding-and-capacity
-data.php.

7. Interim Guidance on Management of Coronavirus Disease
    2019 (COVID-19) in Correctional and Detention Facilities.
    Centers for Disease Control and Prevention. March 27, 2020.
    https://www.cdc.gov/coronavirus/2019-ncov/community
    /correctiondetention/guidance-correctional-detention.html
    (page discontinued).

8. Smith S. COVID-19 in Crowded Mississippi Prisons "a Disaster
    Waiting to Happen." *Mississippi Center for Investigative
    Reporting.* May 16, 2020. https://www.mississippicir.org/news
    /covid-19-in-crowded-mississippi-prisons-a-disaster-waiting
    -to-happen.

9. Shapiro J. Doubling Up Prisoners in "Solitary" Creates
    Deadly Consequences. *North Country Public Radio.*
    March 24, 2016. https://www.northcountrypublicradio.org
    /news/npr/470824303/doubling-up-prisoners-in-solitary
    -creates-deadly-consequences#:~:text=%22We've%20
    done%20this%20utterly,for%20more%20than%2030%20
    years.

10. Expert Report of Homer Venters in Case 4:19-cv-00212
    -MW-MAF, Document 311. United States District Court North-
    ern District of Florida Tallahassee Division. Filed May 28,
    2021. https://www.courtlistener.com/docket/15763248/431/12
    /harvard-v-dixon/.

11. Fonrouge G. Squalid, Crowded Conditions Return to Rikers
    Island Intake Center. *New York Post.* June 14, 2022. https://
    nypost.com/2022/06/14/squalid-crowded-conditions-return
    -to-rikers-island-intake-center/.

12. Expert Report of Homer Venters in Fernandez-Rodriguez v.
    Licon-Vitale. Case 1:20-cv-03315-ER, Document 51. United
    States District Court Southern District of New York. Filed
    May 26, 2020. https://www.fd.org/sites/default/files/covid19
    /bop_jail_policies_and_information/doc_51.pdf.

13. Torres et al. v. Milusnic et al. Case 2:20-cv-04450-CBM-PVC, Document 239-1. United States District Court, Central District of California. Filed May 12, 2021. https://www.lisa -legalinfo.com/wp-content/uploads/2021/07/VentersReport Dkt239-20cv4450.pdf.

14. Interim Guidance on Management of Coronavirus Disease 2019 (COVID-19) in Correctional and Detention Facilities. Updated July 22, 2020. Accessed September 19, 2020. https://www.cdc .gov/coronavirus/2019-ncov/community/correctiondetention /guidance-correctional-detention.html (page discontinued).

15. Interim Guidance on Management of Coronavirus Disease 2019 (COVID-19).

16. Improving Ventilation in Your Home. Centers for Disease Control and Prevention. April 13, 2023. https://www.cdc.gov/coronavirus /2019-ncov/prevent-getting-sick/improving-ventilation-home .html#:~:text=Ventilation%3A%20moves%20air%20into%2C %20out,remove%20them%20from%20the%20air.

17. Expert Report of Homer Venters in Case 4:20-cv-00434. ECF No. 128. United States District Court Eastern District Arkansas. Filed January 14, 2021. https://www.courtlistener .com/docket/17128817/128/frazier-v-graves/; Jewett C, Weber L. Boeing Tested Air Purifiers Like Those Widely Used in Schools and Decided Not to Use Them. *Seattle Times*. June 14, 2021. https://www.seattletimes.com/seattle-news /health/boeing-tested-air-purifiers-like-those-widely-used-in -schools-and-decided-not-to-use-them/; Simpson S. Arkansas Prisons Take Covid Measures; $2M Air-Purification System Among Board-Approved Items. *Arkansas Online*. August 25, 2021. https://www.arkansasonline.com/news/2021/aug/25 /prisons-take-covid-measures/.

18. Gates J. Chris Epps Sentenced to Almost 20 Years. *Clarion Ledger*. May 24, 2017. https://www.clarionledger.com/story /news/2017/05/24/chris-epps-sentencing/341916001/; Amy J. Casino Chips and Prison Contracts: 5 Years Later, Chris Epps Bribery Scheme Still Playing Out. *Clarion Ledger*. August 19, 2019. https://www.clarionledger.com/story/news/politics/2019

/08/19/prison-bribery-scheme-chris-epps-4-la-men-change
-not-guilty-pleas-leblanc-contracts/2048361001/.

19. Kirby J. Nassau County Executive and His Wife Arrested in
Federal Corruption Probe. *New York Magazine.* October 20,
2016. https://nymag.com/intelligencer/2016/10/nassau-county
-executive-arrested-in-federal-corruption-probe.html.

20. Quandt KR, Fenster A. It's All About the Incentives: Why a Call
Home from a Jail in New York State Can Cost 7 Times More
Than the Same Call from the State's Prisons. Prison Policy
Initiative. August 23, 2021. https://www.prisonpolicy.org/blog
/2021/03/23/ny-jail-phones/#:~:text=We%20found%20
that%20the%20majority,pockets%20of%20the%20county%20
government.

21. Ortiz A. Lawsuits Accuse 2 Michigan Jails of Banning Family
Visits to Increase Revenue. *New York Times.* March 28, 2024.
https://www.nytimes.com/2024/03/28/us/jail-visits-ban
-michigan-lawsuit.html; Families of Prisoners Sue Nation's
Largest Providers of Inmate Calling Services for Fixing and
Lying about Prices. Washington Lawyers' Committee for Civil
Rights and Urban Affairs. June 29, 2020. https://www.washlaw
.org/families-of-prisoners-sue-nations-largest-providers-of
-inmate-calling-services-for-fixing-and-lying-about-prices/.

22. Carson EA, Nadel M, Gaes G. Impact of COVID-19 on State
and Federal Prisons, March 2020–February 2021. Bureau of
Justice Statistics. August 2022. https://bjs.ojp.gov/library
/publications/impact-covid-19-state-and-federal-prisons
-march-2020-february-2021; Decarceration and Crime During
COVID-19. ACLU. July 27, 2020. https://www.aclu.org/news
/smart-justice/decarceration-and-crime-during-covid-19.

23. The Civil Rights Litigation Clearinghouse website can be
found at https://clearinghouse.net/about.

INDEX

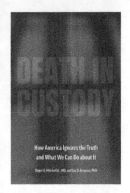
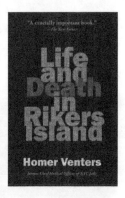
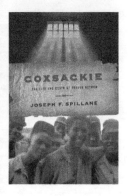